Gender and the Social Construction of Illness

Judith Lorber

Brooklyn College
City University of New York

SAGE PUBLICATIONS

Thousand Oaks ■ London ■ New Delhi

For information:

SAGE Publications, Inc.
2455 Teller Road
Thousand Oaks, California 91320
E-mail: order@sagepub.com

SAGE Publications Ltd.
6 Bonhill Street
London EC2A 4PU
United Kingdom

SAGE Publications India Pvt. Ltd.
M-32 Market
Greater Kailash I
New Delhi 110 048 India

Printed in the United States of America

Library of Congress Cataloging-in-Publication Data

Lorber, Judith.
    Gender and the social construction of illness/Judith Lorber.
        p.   cm. — (Gender lens; vol. 4)
    Includes bibliographical references (p.   ) and index.
    ISBN 0-8039-5813-7 (cloth).—ISBN 0-8039-5814-5 (pbk.)
        1. Social medicine. 2. Sexism in medicine. 3. Women—Health and hygiene—Sociological aspects. 4. Men—Health and hygiene—Sociological aspects. 5. Sex role. 6. Feminist theory.
    I. Title. II. Series.
    RA418.L67   1997   97-4588
    306.4'61—dc21

Acquiring Editor: Peter Labella
Editorial Assistant: Frances Borghi
Production Editor: Sherrise M. Purdum
Production Assistant: Denise Santoyo
Copy Editor: Joyce Kuhn
Typesetter/Designer: Marion Warren
Indexer: Teri Greenberg
Print Buyer: Anna Chin

CONTENTS

For Lorrie and Phyllis,

who have gone through life with me

The current volume presents a gendered analysis of health, illness, and medical care. Judith Lorber uses familiar concepts in medical sociology reconceptualized through a gender lens. The current volume addresses two basic issues. First, the author pays critical attention to the social aspects of the experience of physical illness and resultant medical care. This involves attention to how gender, race, class, ethnicity, and culture influence the experience of symptoms and how such symptoms are treated by the medical establishment. Second, the author uses a gender lens to critically examine the social construction of the knowledge base and underlying assumptions about illness. She critiques the way questions are asked and research priorities set.

Although medical sociologists have addressed these issues in the past, they have usually done so without a gender lens. For medical sociologists, gender has meant women—first, patients and nurses, and then doctors. When medical sociologists have added women to research it has usually meant comparing women's and men's sickness and death rates, differences in behavior and in treatment as patients, behaviors as doctors, and so on. But much of the analysis of the social construction of medical knowledge and beliefs did not incorporate a concern with the social construction of gender.

For feminists who study health and illness, attention to gender has meant concern with the status of women and men in the social order. Feminists have asked why, how, and by whom such normal physiological events as menstruation and menopause have been turned into illnesses and consequently into social problems. They have looked at the gendered dimensions of the hierarchy of medical occupations and what happens when men are nurses and women are doctors. Feminist have also questioned the objectivity and neutrality of scientific findings that come out of a professional world dominated by men.

In this volume, Judith Lorber weaves together medical, sociological, and feminist concerns as she takes a gender lens on health, illness, and medicine. Lorber shows how gender is an integral part of the transformation of physiological symptoms into illness. She reviews sex differences in social epidemiology— rates of illness and longevity—and provides data for the proposition that these are the results of social statuses—race, class, and gender. Premenstrual tension and menopause are discussed at length as examples of the processes by which normal physiological female phenomena become illnesses that denigrate women's social status. Lorber provides an in-depth look at the current AIDS epidemic. The book ends with a proposal for leveling the hierarchies and inequalities in medicine through feminist health care practices and suggests that this would be beneficial for men as well as for women.

We hope this book, and others in the *Gender Lens* series will help the reader develop her or his own "gender lens" to better and more accurately understand our social environments. As sociologists, we believe that an accurate understanding of inequality is a prerequisite for effective social change.

Judith Howard
Barbara Risman
Mary Romero
Joey Sprague
Gender Lens Series Editors

A C K N O W L E D G M E N T S

I would like to thank Mitch Allen, the first *Gender Lens* series editor at Sage, for persuading me to do this book, and the editors of the series—Judy Howard, Barbara Risman, Mary Romero, and Joey Sprague—for their encouragement and advice. I am grateful to Elianne Riska, who suggested the theoretical work on the social construction of the body; Edward J. Farrell, Jr., who supplied the life expectancy statistics; and Joyce Wallace and Brenda Seals, who reviewed the chapter on AIDS.

For their very helpful critique of the writing as it went through its drafts, my thanks go to the members of my writing group—Maren Carden, Susan Farrell, Eileen Moran, and Barbara Katz Rothman—and to Barbara Risman, my Gender Lens *madrina*, Peter Labella, the current series editor at Sage, and Joey Sprague. I would also like to thank Judi Addelston and the reference librarians at the Mina Reese CUNY Graduate School Library for their indispensable literature searches.

Parts of this book were adapted from *Paradoxes of Gender* (Yale University Press, 1994).

Judith Lorber
New York City

CHAPTER 1

Gender and the Social Construction of Illness

Overview

> It has been assumed that anything and everything worth understanding
> can be explained or interpreted within the assumptions of modern
> science. Yet there is another world hidden from the consciousness of
> science—the world of emotions, feelings, political values; of the
> individual and collective unconscious; of social and historical
> particularity. . . . Part of the project of feminism is to reveal the
> relationship between these two worlds—how each shapes and forms the
> other. (Harding 1986:245)

We usually consider physical health as a state in which people can do what they
have to do and want to do, and illness as something that disturbs the physiological equilibrium of the body. But what we actually experience as illness is a
disturbance of our social lives so that we cannot go about our usual pursuits, a
situation which may or may not be the result of actual bodily dysfunctioning.
The perception that something is wrong and the guesses as to the cause are
always experienced in a social context. Thus, a homemaker in a poor community
said when asked to define illness,

> I wish I really knew what you meant about being sick. Sometimes I felt so bad
> I could curl up and die, but had to go on because the kids had to be taken care
> of, and besides, we didn't have the money to spend for the doctor—how could
> I be sick? . . . How do you know when you're sick, anyway? Some people can
> go to bed almost any time with anything, but most of us can't be sick—even
> when we need to be. (Koos 1954:30)[1]

In every society, the symptoms, pains, and weaknesses called illness are
shaped by cultural and moral values, experienced through interaction with
members of one's immediate social circle and visits to health care professionals,
and influenced by beliefs about health and illness. The result is a transformation
of physiological symptoms into diagnoses or illness names, socially appropriate
illness behavior, and heroic and stigmatized social statuses. This transformation
is heavily influenced by power differences and moral judgments. Not all patients

1

(nor, for that matter, health care workers) are equal—gender, racial ethnic category, social class, sexual orientation, and type of illness produce differences in social worth and social power. These power differences permeate research priorities, treatment modes, and the production of medical knowledge.

In Western societies, the culture and language of illness and medical knowledge comes from science—"medical science" is the way we talk about what doctors know and do. Other health care professionals, such as nurses, are also trained in medical science. The scientific base of medicine uses a *biomedical model* of disease. This model assumes that disease is a deviation from normal biological functioning, that diseases have specific causes that can be located in the ill person's body, that diseases have the same symptoms and outcome in any social situation, and that medicine is a socially neutral science (Mishler 1981). Critics of this model have shown that what is normal depends on who is being compared to whom, that many diseases have social and environmental causes, that illness rates and severity vary from place to place, and that the values underlying medical research, practice, theories, and knowledge are deeply biased by the practice situations and the social characteristics of the dominant group of medical professionals—physicians.[2]

Critical medical sociologists provided ample evidence of race and class biases in Western medicine, and feminists added gender to the list.[3] They argued that medical norms were based on white, middle-class men's bodies; therefore, all women who menstruated, got pregnant, and went through menopause were sick. They showed that physicians did not take women's daily lives into account when considering the causes of diseases or prescribing treatment. And most crucial, they challenged scientific claims to universality.[4] How could medical science be trusted, they asked, when so few women were scientists, when the diseases that killed men were the first priority in research, when women were not included in clinical trials, when women's bodies and experiences were ignored as data, and when women's second-class status permeated their treatment as patients?

A complete analysis of health and illness as social phenomena must include gender. My intent in this book is to show how gender, in conjunction with the socially constructed categories of race, ethnicity, class, and sexual orientation, creates different risks and protections for physical illnesses, produces different behavior when ill, elicits different responses in health care personnel, affects the social worth of patients, and influences priorities of treatment, research, and financing.

I will concentrate on problems that are located in the body, such as infections, cancers, or nonfunctioning limbs or senses, and physical processes, such as menstruation and menopause, that in Western society have been transformed into illnesses. These bodily manifestations are often influenced by feelings of stress, anxiety, and depression, but the symptoms or cause are primarily physical. The *context*, however, is *social*, and social contexts are usually gendered—they have different effects on women and men.

Researchers first sought for direct links between emotions, particularly stress, and illness but soon found that the path was more complex and indirect (Thoits 1995). People in stressful situations, such as demanding jobs or family conflict, often drink and smoke more, eat too much, drive recklessly, and in general neglect their health. Their behavior puts them at risk for heart attacks, lung and liver cancer, and automobile accidents. Their emotions can therefore be said to have an indirect health effect. But the situations they are in are stressful because of their social contexts—a working-class person who is supervising other workers may be getting too little respect from them and too little authority from those above; a single parent may have the double responsibility of child care and economic support. Thus, the path between emotions and illness starts with a structural or institutional context that produces a stressful social situation for an individual who then engages in risky behavior that can have detrimental effects on health (Link and Phelan 1995). Economic resources, coping strategies, and social supports help buffer the individual from the negative effects of stress.

Gender differences here are both direct and statistical. Divorce and separation tend to produce more risky behavior in men, such as drinking, and more emotional reactions in women, such as depression (Aneshensel, Rutter, and Lachenbruch 1991; Horwitz, White, and Howell-White 1996). The social context for middle-class American single men is that they are likely to be looking for dates in bars and at parties; for single women, facing the dating scene in their late 30s and 40s (or older) can be thoroughly depressing. In contrast, both men and women who are single parents of small children juggle myriad responsibilities and get too little sleep and exercise and eat poorly. They are prone to stomachaches, colds, and other minor but bothersome gastrointestinal and upper respiratory problems (Gove 1984). The lack of social supports for single parents in the United States has a gender-neutral impact, but since many more women than men are likely to be single parents, the statistical outcome is that women are more frequently sick and absent from work.

The *body in its social context*, therefore, is this book's subject.

Gender and the Social
Transformation of the Body

The framework for this gender lens on illness and health is the *transformation of the body through gendered social practices.*[5] These practices start before birth—what a pregnant woman eats, what prenatal technology and care are available to her, what her family and educational and economical status are, and what social worth a child of a woman of her racial ethnic group, economic status, and family background is likely to have all affect the fetus, infant, and growing child as profoundly as genetic inheritance. Social practices produce social bodies all through life and death—and beyond (consider how corpses are handled). Because gender is embedded in the major social organizations of society, such as the economy, the family, politics, and the medical and legal systems, it has a major impact on how the women and men of different social groups are treated in all sectors of life, including health and illness, getting born and dying. Gender is thus one of the most significant factors in the transformation of physical bodies into social bodies.[6]

For example, in Western culture, dieting, breast enhancement, and face lifts are ways that women and girls change their bodies to fit an ideal of feminine beauty, while men and boys lift weights and get hair transplants to mold their bodies to a masculine ideal (Bordo 1993; Davis 1995; Gullette 1993). These practices may lead to illnesses, such as eating disorders, infections, and systemic damage from leaking silicone implants, but by themselves, they are not considered abnormal in our culture because they are responses to accepted views of how women's and men's bodies should look. The transformation of bodies that might be less differentiable into bodies that are markedly masculine and feminine is typical of the pressures of gender. Even competitive women bodybuilders downplay their size, use makeup, wear their hair long and blond, and emphasize femininity in posing by using "dance, grace, and creativity"; otherwise, they don't win competitions (Mansfield and McGinn 1993). Similarly, if men football players don't ignore injuries and pain and use their bodies aggressively on the field, their masculinity is impugned by coaches and fellow players (Messner 1992).

The Social Construction of Illness

Although it is located in the body, illness as a social experience goes far beyond physiology. For patients and health care professionals, it involves all the patterns of social life—interlocking social roles, power and conflict, social statuses, networks of family and friends, bureaucracies and organizations, social control, ideas of moral worth, aspects of work and occupations, definitions of reality, and the production of knowledge (Brown 1995). A broken leg may be a simple fracture, but it is experienced entirely differently by a professional athlete, for whom it is a career stopper, and an office worker, for whom it is an annoying temporary encumbrance. Two illnesses, say pneumonia and gonorrhea, may be easily treated by antibiotics and quite curable, but the social effects of pneumonia are far different from the social consequences of gonorrhea. If you have had gonorrhea, you may want to keep it a secret in a physical examination for a job. If you have had pneumonia, you may have to stay home from work if you have a bad cold, but you won't keep it a secret when asked about previous serious illnesses. In one society, the physical cessation of menstruation puts the women into a revered status, in another, in a status of lesser social worth.

Because illness is socially constructed, physicians and patients may see the same set of symptoms (or lack of them) entirely differently. Physicians tend to look first for visible physical symptoms or clear test results. For them, the ideal illness situation is one that produces an unambiguous diagnosis with effective treatment that cures the disease by removing the symptoms or that restores the patient to more or less normal functioning. For patients, modified ability to conduct their lives—chronic but treatable conditions—is a considerably different situation than complete cure. A cure restores them to their former roles; a chronic condition forces them to modify those roles and establish new patterns of behavior. Similarly, what the physician may see as unavoidable side effects from necessary treatment, the patient may experience as unwarranted increased pain or discomfort, stress, and financial cost. Patients who feel the physician is at fault may sue for malpractice.

The social construction of illness influences the search for causes. If symptoms are not visible or test results are ambiguous, the physician may infer a psychological cause, which the patient may or may not accept. Or the physician may insist that the patient is exaggerating symptoms or even faking them, which the patient may vociferously deny. A physician may give a patient a "clean bill of health" based on no significant pathology or abnormality, but the patient may persist in worrying that something is still wrong. A nurse practitioner might discuss the social aspects of the patient's problem more than a physician is likely to (Fisher 1995).

Patients with visible symptoms, clear test results, and an unambiguous diagnosis may face moral criticism or avoidance, both by professionals and laypeople, if their illness is sexually transmitted, the result of substance abuse, or highly infectious. This stigma may never leave them, even if they are restored to practically normal functioning. Conversely, patients with severe disabilities, chronic conditions, or terminal illness, if they meet their situation with good grace—stoicism, cheerfulness, and gratitude for care—may be called heroic or saintly.

Gender and Illness

As a social phenomenon, illness has to be gendered because gender is one of the most important statuses in any society. Gender is also socially constructed. Girls and boys are taught their society's expectations of appropriate behavior; they grow up to enact their society's gendered social roles. Gender is a social institution that patterns interaction in everyday life and in major social organizations (Lorber 1994). Gender impacts on illness through economic circumstances, work and family responsibilities, lifestyle choices, social interaction with family members and other intimates, and interactions with health professionals.[7] For health care workers, including physicians, occupations and specializations are gendered (Lorber 1984).

The juxtaposition of gender and illness presents two major problems: sex differences versus gender differences and between-group differences versus within-group differences.

All human beings are physiologically similar, but females and males also have clear physiological differences. However, beyond the reproductive system, it is not known how extensive —or minimal—these sex differences are.[8] According to Lois Verbrugge (1989a), who has worked on the problem for many years,

> The vulnerabilities and the resistances that males and females typically re-
> ceive at conception, or how aging processes and social exposures alter the size
> and character of one's given robustness, are not known. The single greatest
> need in population studies of sex differences in health and mortality is
> operational measures of that biological substrate. (p. 296)

⅄ It is extremely difficult to isolate basic biological sex differences because biology, physiology, genetic inheritance, and hormonal input always occur in and are shaped by social and environmental contexts (Lorber 1993b). Better known are the social factors that cause women to be prone to more minor illnesses during their lifetime, to see health care professionals more often, and to live longer and men to be vulnerable to physical traumas, medical crises, and early death. These are *gender differences*—the differences that emerge from social interaction and social status in complex interplay with biology, genetic inheritance, hormones, and physiology.

There are also racial, ethnic, educational, occupational, and social class divisions among women and men. Comparisons of "women" and "men" often do not do justice to this variation:

> If we turn to those conditions that afflict both men and women—the majority of all diseases and health problems—we must keep two things simultaneously in mind. First are the differences and similarities among diverse groups of women [and men], second are the differences and similarities between women and men. (Fee and Krieger 1994b:18)

For health care providers, work setting and professional norms have important effects that can override gender. For example, the behavior of men and women doctors sometimes reflects their professional status and sometimes their gender, and it is important to look at both aspects to understand their relationships with patients (Lorber 1985). Among nurses, most of whom are women, race and ethnicity stratify the profession, with better educated and upwardly mobile registered nurses mostly white and licensed practical nurses and nurses' aides predominantly Blacks and Latinas (Glazer 1991; Glenn 1992).

The Social Context

The social context is an integral part of any illness. From the recognition and attention to symptoms through actions while sick to coping with recovery or a chronic condition or dying, all of patients' social characteristics have an effect. This effect is shaped by their social networks, their work and financial status, their family obligations, and the medical care systems and values of their society. As medical care systems change, so does the behavior of patients and health care professionals.

For the greater part of the 20th century, American medicine was practiced by physicians working alone in their offices, visiting their patients in hospitals, and collecting a fee for their services (Starr 1982). Patients and physicians negotiated with each other directly, but the physician had all the power and prestige. Patients tended to see physicians of their own race and religion but not their own gender, since women studying medicine were kept to a quota of about 5-6 percent in medical schools that admitted them and in hospitals where they did their clinical training (Walsh 1977). One medical school for women survived the professionalization of medicine in the early 1900s—the Women's Medical College of Pennsylvania—but no all-women's hospitals did. Because of religious quotas, Catholic and Jewish men physicians trained in and put their patients into hospitals supported by Catholic and Jewish charities (Solomon 1961). African American and Hispanic physicians went to federally funded medical schools and used mostly publicly funded hospitals or community-based clinics (Hine 1985; Moldow 1987). Nurses were strictly under physicians' orders (Reverby 1987). Native American and other indigenous healers, although they had many clients in their communities, were not considered legitimate health care workers.

Today, the structure of medical training and practice is much closer to that of other countries with Western medical systems.[9] Women physicians of all racial ethnic groups make up half or more of most medical school classes, but medical specialties are not evenly gender integrated. Nurse practitioners and nurse midwives are responsible for their own patients. More nurses and nursing administrators are men. Native and alternative health providers, such as acupuncturists and nutritional specialists, are paid for by health insurance. The major change in the structure of medical care in the United States is the expansion of health maintenance organizations (HMOs), where the provider is paid by a third party (insurance agency or the government), where the patient's choice of physicians and hospitals is often restricted, and where the physician's choice of treatments and medications is confined to what the payer allows. Physicians have lost prestige and authority, but patients have not gained any power in the medical encounter (Freidson 1989). The third party in the negotiation is the payer, a large, for-profit or government bureaucracy that tries to develop one-size-fits-all rules. In such a system, the essence of illness—its diversified social context—is suppressed. It is from this context that the inevitable conflicts over health care are likely to come.[10]

In sum, although all human beings experience the universal physical phenomena of birth, growth, illness, aging, and death, and each individual's experiences of these phenomena is particular, between these universals and these particulars are the similarities that come out of membership in social groups —women and men of various racial categories, ethnicities, and economic classes living at different times and in different places. Their social location produces their patterns of health and illness behavior, with the actions of professionals they encounter in seeking help and the organizational structure of the medical system they must deal with in getting treatment equally important in shaping their experiences as patients.

Overview of the Book

This book's focus is a *gender analysis* of the transformation of physiological symptoms into the social reality we call illness. A gender analysis shows how gender is built into almost every aspect of illness in modern society: risks of and protections from different diseases, the perception and response of the patient to symptoms, the organization and delivery of health care, the politics of diagnosis, funding priorities, the questions asked by clinical and scientific researchers, and the knowledge and meaning of diseases and their treatment. Each chapter examines major concepts in medical sociology through a gender lens perspective. These areas are *social epidemiology and risks of disease; the doctor-nurse-patient relationship and the sick role; the politics of diagnosis and "woman troubles" (premenstrual syndrome and menopause); and the social construction of AIDS—a modern plague.* The concluding chapter discusses ways in which the recommendations of *feminist health care* can be applied to everyone.

Chapter 2, "Women Get Sicker, But Men Die Quicker," explains epidemiological rates of death and illness in terms of women's and men's *sociocultural risk factors.* These factors are a combination of gender norms, racial ethnic group membership, economic status, age, and social relationships. The social environment and social practices in which risk factors are embedded materially transform bodies and make them vulnerable to or protect them from the causes of illness. Epidemiological statistics are affected more by social factors than physiology. Take one of the obvious differences between females and males—females get pregnant and give birth and males do not. Before Western medicine provided the means to prevent and cure infections, many young women died in childbirth; in prosperous communities today, childbearing women live much longer than men. In societies where there is little food and medicine and boys get what little there is, more girl babies than boy babies die, even though girls are physically hardier than boys as infants.

Ideally, the combination of sociocultural risk factors ought to be estimated for individuals, with their risks minimized and protections maximized. Social epidemiology, however, estimates group factors. Rates then depend on how these groups are constructed—how they are divided by race and ethnicity, gender, social class, place of residence, religion, and so on. The way social factors are categorized produces differential rates of illness and estimations of proneness to different diseases (Jones, Snider, and Warren 1996; Krieger 1996).

These statistics about gender differences in health and illness (morbidity) and birth and death rates (mortality) not only reflect social processes, they are also social constructions. Social epidemiological statistics are influenced by what questions are asked and how the answers are categorized as well as by the reliability of techniques of information gathering and measurement. Unless women and men of different races, religions, and social classes are included in a sample, researchers have no way of making socially useful comparisons of health status, health practices, and risk-taking behavior. These statistics are usually not value free; priorities are set by those who have the power and resources to get answers to the questions of importance to them. One might say that what counts gets counted.

For the past 25 years, gender, racial ethnic group, social class, and religious affiliation have been viewed as affecting health through *social advantages and disadvantages,* not through physiological differences (Fee and Krieger 1994b). Different groups of people are *at risk* for different kinds of diseases because of where they live, what they eat, what kind of health care they have access to, and whether they have social supports in times of difficulty (Link and Phelan 1995).

In addition, varied patterns of *risk taking* protect or endanger people throughout their lives.

In modern countries with Westernized medical systems, younger men are prone to traumatic injuries, homicide, and suicide and older men to life-threatening cardiovascular diseases. Women of all ages show higher rates of minor illnesses of all kinds, yet live longer. But "the quality of life of those extra years is exceptionally burdened by cancer, particularly of the breast, lung, and colon, by heart disease and stroke, osteoporosis, Alzheimer's disease, depression and social isolation, and general frailty" (Healy 1991:275). Although more men than women have died of AIDS-related pathologies, the rate of HIV infection among heterosexual women is climbing, and there is some evidence that they die more quickly once infected (Melnick et al. 1994). These epidemiological statistics are not solely the result of the physiological differences between males and females but are also the outcome of gendered family roles, lifestyles, occupations, and the norms and expectations of masculinity and femininity. These social factors, the processes that make male and female bodies vulnerable to illnesses and to dying at different ages, are reflected in morbidity and mortality rates.

Symptoms do not make a woman or man a patient—seeking professional help does. An important aspect of the patient's experience in any kind of illness is interaction with professionals, who are the source of expertise and authority in medical settings. Chapter 3, "The Doctor Knows Best," analyzes the interactive behavior of women and men doctors, nurses, and patients in hospitals, offices, and clinics. The gendered power differences in the triad produce the norm expectations each participant has for each other along with the conflicts and negotiations over diagnoses and treatment. The frame for the analysis is how the medical system structures patient-professional interaction in *the sick role*. This role connects the patient's lived experience with the medical system, the state of knowledge about the disease, and the social statuses of all concerned.

In the *doctor-nurse-patient relationship*, power differences between patients and physicians and between physicians and other health care workers mean that physicians set the agenda for taking a history of symptoms, and patients' "lifeworld" concerns may simply go unheard (Mishler 1984). Physician also have the authority to diagnose patients' problems and prescribe what they consider appropriate treatment. Other health care workers take their orders from the physician in charge of the case. Differences of opinion are suppressed by the hierarchy of patient-nurse-physician, which is reinforced when the patient and the nurse are women and the physician is a man and is weakened when the physician is a woman and the nurse and the patient are men.

Whether the physician is a women or a man influences how much attention is paid to women's and men's presenting complaints, especially what kind of tests are ordered (Franks and Clancy 1993; Kreuter et al. 1995). Women's symptoms are more likely to be labeled psychosomatic by men physicians, who are more likely than women physicians to prescribe tranquilizers to them than to men patients with similar symptoms (Ettorre, Klaukka, and Riska 1994; Taggart et al. 1993). Nurse practitioners are trained to look for the interaction of psychosocial factors with physiological symptoms and treat them simultaneously (Fisher 1995). Thus, the interpretation of the same symptoms can be quite different and depend on the gender, training, and experience of the health care provider and the gender and other social characteristics of the patient. This interaction of women and men patients and the structural position of women and men health care personnel creates gendered sick roles.[11]

Different types of sick roles have different social consequences, but sociologically, all illnesses are considered *deviance* because the symptoms make it impossible for people to pursue their normal social roles. People with such symptoms are not blamed for staying home from work or school or not doing home chores, but they are held responsible for seeking professional help and cooperating with treatment in an effort to return to normal. Some illnesses do not allow a return to normal—they are chronic, permanently disabling, or degenerative. Others, such as sexually transmitted diseases, are stigmatizing, and so, even after recovery, the person's social identity is contaminated if the previous illness is revealed.[12]

With other conditions, such as *premenstrual tension and menopause,* the process of interpretation and definition of the situation creates a disorder where none may actually be present. In these situations, the patient and the physician may be in disagreement as to the presence and severity of the condition. It is only when the physician and the patient agree that you have an uncontested diagnosis of "true illness" or "true wellness." That is, without the doctor's validation, the patient's version of the situation is not considered official. When signs of disease are found at a checkup, even if the patient feels well, he or she is considered ill. If the patient claims symptoms and the physician finds no signs of disease, the patient may be labeled a hypochondriac, malingerer, or hysteric. If the physician constructs a syndrome with a name out of diffuse symptoms, as with many so-called "women's troubles," treatment may be prescribed for what the woman might otherwise consider a natural condition.[13]

Chapter 4, "If a Situation Is Defined as Real . . . ," examines the ways in which premenstrual tension and menopausal mood swings are socially and medically constructed. The transformation of symptoms individually experienced at different points in women's procreative life cycle into medically recognized physiological and psychological syndromes clearly illustrates the social construction of illness. Some women might pay little attention to premenstrual tension, menstrual cramps, and menopausal hot flashes, while others might need treatment for them. But if these occurrences are routinely labeled illnesses by the medical profession, then all women will often be considered "sick" or not able to function normally. The part that medicine as a social institution plays in legitimizing appropriate behavior in women can be seen as a form of *social control.*[14]

When an illness assumes epidemic proportions and its spread has moral overtones, the cultural, religious, and ideological values of a society override individual factors in how chronically ill people are treated. Chapter 5, "A Modern Plague," takes illness into the moral realm of social identities contaminated by *stigmatized diseases.* AIDS (acquired immunodeficiency syndrome) is an epidemic imbued with gender, sexuality, class, race, and ethnicity. AIDS is very much affected by gender in its transmission and treatment (Campbell 1990; Cooper 1995). Its physical ravages and social aspects differ significantly for women and men of different racial ethnic groups, economic strata, and sexual orientations. The discourse and dynamics around AIDS show how sickness is reflective of cultural views of women and men, homosexuals and heterosexuals, poor and rich, people of color and whites, and "foreigners" and "natives." Patients are supposed to be treated, not punished, but moral issues and the fear of contagion create conditions where patients may be controlled in an effort to control the disease. Other patients may lack care or not be able to obtain necessary treatment because they are not defined as sick enough—or as too far gone to do anything for.

How HIV-positive status and the symptoms of AIDS are reacted to and treated reflect heterosexual, bisexual, and homosexual relationships; the constellation of patient, practitioners, and lay caretakers; community attitudes; cultural values; and the politics of medical bureaucracies and government agencies. AIDS has been a feared epidemic because there is as yet no vaccination against HIV infection and no cure for a severely damaged immune system. Those who are known to be HIV positive or to show the signs of full-blown AIDS have been stigmatized for their sexual practices or drug use and out of fear of contagion from their semen, blood, or saliva. From negotiations over condom use between sexual partners to allocation of funds for research and treatment by national and international agencies, AIDS literally and figuratively embodies the material, experiential, and symbolic gendered construction of illness.

Chapter 6, "Treating Social Bodies in Social Worlds," looks at the conflict between the ways that professionals and laypeople define medical reality and proposes an alternative: *feminist health care.* This perspective sees the patient and the health care professional as equals in the medical encounter. The doctor or nurse knows more about illnesses and their treatment in general, but the patient knows more about her or his particular case. Feminist health care advocates recommend that before the professionals apply general medical science, they should understand patients' social and environmental contexts and also patients' history of the particular disease (Candib 1995). When professionals prescribe a course of treatment, they should tell patients not only what the risks and side effects are but also advise as to the advantages and disadvantages of other courses of treatment and nontreatment. Then patients should decide what they want to do and expect the continued support and help of the professionals, even if the professionals' first choice for treatment was rejected.

Feminist health care is for all patients—men as well as women, older children as well as adults. As a way of providing medical services, it must be taught in medical schools, reinforced in clinical training, and built into day-to-day practices by organizational policies that encourage enough time for listening and payment for diverse types of treatment. This is an idealistic goal, but if it is shared by both the providers and the consumers of care, it could go a long way in empowering the most powerless members of these overlapping groups—the poor, the young, people of color, the less educated, and women.

Notes

1. Also see Horton 1984 and Popay 1992.

2. Freidson 1970a, 1970b; Mishler 1981, 1984; Waitzkin 1983, 1991; and Wright and Treacher 1982.

3. For overall critiques, see Fisher 1986; Lorber 1975a; Martin [1987] 1992; Todd 1989; Ruzek 1978; and Zimmerman 1987. For a summary of the contribution of sociologists, see Auerbach and Figert 1995.

4. For feminist critiques of science, see Birke 1986; Harding 1986, 1991; Hubbard 1990; Keller 1985; Longino 1990; and Schiebinger 1989.

5. For theories of the social body, see Featherstone, Hepworth, and Turner 1991; Gallagher and Laqueur 1987; O'Neill 1985, 1989; Scheper-Hughes and Lock 1987; Shilling 1993; and Turner 1984, 1992.

6. Bordo 1993; Butler 1993; Connell 1995; Hubbard 1990; Jordanova 1989; Laqueur 1990; and Martin [1987] 1992.

7. An early study, still in print, is Ehrenreich and English 1973a. For current studies, see Bair and Cayleff 1993; Bayne-Smith 1996; Dan 1994; Doyal 1995; Fee and Krieger 1994a; Kristiansen 1989; Lewin and Oleson 1985; Muller 1990; Ratcliff 1989; Sabo and Gordon 1995a, 1995b; Santow 1995; and White 1990.

8. The differentiation of the sexes is not as categorically dual as is usually thought. Male and female genitalia develop from the same fetal tissue, and so, because of various genetic and hormonal inputs, at least 1 in 1,000 infants are born with ambiguous genitalia (Fausto-Sterling 1993). An anomaly common enough to be found in several feminine-looking women at every major international sports competition is the existence of XY chromosomes that have not produced male anatomy or physiology because of other genetic input (Grady 1992). As for hormones, recent research suggests that testosterone and other androgens are as important to normal development in females as in males, and that in both, testosterone is converted to estrogen in the brain (Angier 1994, 1995).

9. For other countries, see Lorber 1984 and Riska and Wegar 1993a, 1993b.

10. In 1996, public and political pressure forced health insurers to allow mothers of newborns to stay in the hospital 48 hours rather than 24. The reasons were both medical and social: Newborns need more observation to make sure there are no developing problems, and women need the rest and care they are unlikely to get at home. In contrast, in Israel, government health insurance pays for two weeks in new-mother centers because Orthodox Jewish women have many children close together.

11. Fisher 1986, 1995; Lorber 1975b, 1985; Scully [1980] 1994; Sherwin 1992; Todd 1989; and West 1984.

12. The conceptualizations of illness as deviance and the sick role as legitimated deviance or as stigmatized were formulated by Parsons 1951 and Freidson 1970a.

13. Abplanalp 1983; Callahan 1993; Guinan 1988; Laws 1983; Laws, Hey, and Egan 1985; Lock 1993; McCrea 1986; Parlee 1994; Rittenhouse 1991; Taylor 1995; Voda, Dinnerstein, and O'Donnell 1982; Yankauskas 1990; and Zita 1988.

14. The medicalization of "bad" behavior, such as drinking and drug taking, can be seen as a form of social control over men (see Conrad and Schneider 1992).

CHAPTER 2

Women Get Sicker, But Men Die Quicker

Social Epidemiology

> In any gender-dichotomized society, the fact that we are born biologically female or male means that our environments will be different: we will live different lives. Because our biology and how we live are dialectically related and build on one another, we cannot vary gender and hold the environment constant. (Hubbard 1990:128)

There is a saying in epidemiology—"women get sicker, but men die quicker." It is a succinct way of summing up the illness and death rates of women and men in modern industrialized societies. In industrialized countries, in the early years of the 20th century, women outlived men only by two to three years; today, women live almost seven years longer (Stillion 1995). Racial differences increase these gender differences. In the United States, although life expectancy for a white infant born in the early 1990s is almost seven years longer for a girl than for a boy, for Black infants, the difference is nine years (Kranczer 1995). The combined racial and sex difference between the longest life expectancy (white girls) and the shortest (Black boys) is almost 15 years (see Table 2.1). Black women and men not only die earlier, but are prone to more illnesses and physical traumas throughout their lives than white women and men. Paradoxically, although white women have the longest life expectancy, they have more illnesses than white men do throughout their adult lives (Verbrugge 1985, 1989a, 1989b). Although women as well as men are subject to heart diseases, cancers, and other life-threatening physical problems, on the whole, women live longer than men in industrialized countries because men get the killer diseases earlier (Verbrugge 1990).

In societies where women's social status is very low, their life expectancy is lower than in industrialized countries because of a combination of social factors: eating last and eating less, complications of frequent childbearing and sexually transmitted diseases because they have no power to demand abstinence or condom use, infections and hemorrhages following genital mutilation, neglect of symptoms of illness until severe, and restricted access to modern health care (Santow 1995; see Table 2.2). The relationship between women's health and their

TABLE 2.1

1993 Life Expectancy (in years) at Birth in the United States, by Sex and Race

	Sex		
Race	*Female*	*Male*	*Sex Difference*
All	78.9	72.1	6.8
White	79.5	73.0	6.5
Black	73.7	64.7	9.0
Racial Difference	5.8	8.3	14.8

SOURCE: Kranczer 1995, Table 2, based on data from the National Center for Health Statistics.

social status is starkly demonstrated by how care is allocated within the family in many traditional societies:

> A lower-status individual, such as a young female, was likely to be treated only with home remedies; when assistance was sought outside the household it was more likely to be from a traditional than a modern therapist. A higher-status individual, such as a male of almost any age or an adult mother of sons, was likely to be taken directly to a private medical practitioner. (Santow 1995:154)

Illness and death rates are not linear or uniformly progressive. Because of a combination of social and environmental factors, life expectancy rates for Russian men have declined from 65.5 years in 1991 to 57.3 years in 1995 (Specter 1995). When a woman moves to another country, her risk of dying of breast cancer gradually changes, for the better or worse, to match the risk in her new place of residence (Kliewer and Smith 1995; Ziegler 1993).

The social epidemiologist's task is to explain these variances in *morbidity* (rates of illness) and *mortality* (rates of death) and to tease out the fundamental causes that produce persistent group differences. Some of these are genetic and physiological and some are social. For example, sickle cell anemia and breast cancer cluster in different racial ethnic groups, but access to knowledge, healthy environments, and up-to-date treatment cluster by social class:

> The reason is that resources like knowledge, money, power, prestige, and social connectedness are transportable from one situation to another, and as health-related situations change, those who command the most resources are best able to avoid risks, diseases, and consequences of disease. (Link and Phelan 1995:87)

Morbidity and mortality rates are useful for policy recommendations only when accompanied by data on social factors, such as economic resources, access

Table 2.2

Male-Female Life Expectancy Rates (in years) for Developed and Developing
Countries, 1990-1995

Region	Male Life Expectancy	Female Life Expectancy	Female-Male Ratio
World	62.7	66.7	106.4
Developed	71.0	78.0	109.9
Developing	61.1	63.9	104.6
Africa	51.4	54.6	106.2
North America	72.7	79.4	109.2
Latin America[a]	65.2	70.9	108.2
Asia[b]	63.6	66.1	103.9
Europe	71.9	78.5	109.2
Former USSR	65.7	74.7	113.7
Oceania[c]	69.9	75.6	108.2

SOURCE: World Health Organization 1995:60.
a. Includes Mexico.
b. Excludes Japan.
c. Excludes Australia and New Zealand.

to health services, community supports, and cultural values. What Nancy Krieger (1996) calls "ecosocial theory"

> asks how we literally incorporate, biologically, social relations (such as those of social class, race/ethnicity, and gender) into our bodies, thereby focusing on who and what drives population patterns of health, disease, and well-being. (p. 135)

The rates of illness and death that are used to assess the health of groups of people are themselves influenced by social factors. For example, reports of sudden infant death syndrome (SIDS) are more common where mothers are poor, have little education, and are from disadvantaged racial ethnic groups. Biological or medical models predict a random distribution over social classes. The high death rates for children of lower socioeconomic status can be interpreted two ways—either (a) social factors, such as poverty, are more important than biological causes, or (b) deaths to poor infants are attributed to SIDS more often than with children from more affluent families (Nam, Eberstein, and Deeb 1989). In either case, social factors are significant, but their effects are quite different. SIDS may be more prevalent among lower socioeconomic classes because of social factors, or it may be just as prevalent among middle and upper classes but be more often reported as a cause of death for a child in a poor family because no one investigates further for other causes.

Another measurement problem in social epidemiology influenced by social factors is how illness rates are constructed: Is it by days off from work, visits to health care professionals, hospital days, medication use, or self-assessment? Women are likely to take more days off, see physicians and other health care workers more often, use more medication, and assess themselves as sicker. That is, women are more likely to attend to minor symptoms than men are for a variety of reasons, among them familiarity with the health care system through reproductive needs. Men are encouraged from childhood to be stoical and so are not likely to see a doctor for nonserious health problems. When they do get sick, they are likely to have more and longer hospital visits. Thus, by epidemiological measures, women are sicker than men most of their adult lives, but the health behavior that produces their high illness rates probably increases their longevity. According to Lois Verbrugge (1985), "Women's greater health care in early years diminishes the severity of their problems compared to same age men, and it ultimately helps extend their lives" (p. 173). Women are not more fragile physically than men, just more self-protective of their health.

Still another social epidemiological issue is immediate and proximate cause of death. The most immediate cause for an 85-year-old woman may be pneumonia, a frequent cause of death in the elderly, but long-term causes may be just as significant. These might be poor nutrition, poor housing, and no support services. Or the causes of death might be multiple. Drinking and smoking combined with high blood pressure, which are frequently reactions to poverty and lack of opportunities for advancement, can precipitate a fatal stroke or heart attack. According to Robert Staples (1995),

> Black men suffer a disproportionate burden of illness. The drug and alcoholism rate for blacks, for example, is about four times higher than whites. Whereas black men suffer higher rates of diabetes, strokes and a variety of chronic illnesses, they are also at the mercy of public hospitals, and, therefore, are the first victims of government cutbacks. When they do go to a hospital, they are more likely to receive inadequate treatment. (p. 123)

So what did a particular Black man die from?

Social factors are not easily teased apart for any group.[1] Women tend to have more non-life-threatening illnesses because of the stresses of routinized jobs, child care, the care of elderly parents, and the "double day" of work and housework (Bird and Fremont 1991; Muller 1990; Ross and Bird 1994; Verbrugge 1986). Men are more prone to chronic and life-threatening diseases, such as heart attacks, because of their lifestyle and, to a lesser extent, their occupations (Helgeson 1995; Waldron 1995). They are also more at risk for traumas, accidents, and homicide because they are more likely to get into dangerous situations (Stillion 1995; Veevers and Gee 1986). Women are more likely to attempt suicide, but men are more likely to succeed at it because they use deadlier methods (Canetto 1992; World Health Organization 1995). Married men tend to be healthier mentally and physically than married women, but they have a worse time physically and mentally for about six months after a divorce, separation, or being widowed

(Farberow et al. 1992; Gove 1984) or until they find another woman to look after their physical and emotional needs.

The statistical patterns of morbidity and mortality—who gets sick with what and who dies when from what—are outcomes of individual behavior shaped by cultural and social factors, such as availability of clean water and good food, access to medical knowledge and technology, and protection from environmental pollution, occupational traumas, and social hazards like war, violent crime, rape, battering, and genital mutilation. For the individual, health is as much affected by combined social statuses (gender, race, ethnic group, social class, occupation, and place of residence) as by personal choices (Calnan 1986; Staples 1995; Stillion 1995; Waldron 1995). Indeed, individual behavior is heavily circumscribed by social statuses—not everyone chooses health risks; for some people, health risks are built into their daily lives.[2] On a broader social system level, rates of illness and death are significantly affected by the behavior of health care providers, the policies of health care institutions and agencies, and the financial support of state and national governments for research and treatment (McKinlay 1996).

Because social factors are so intertwined, gender cannot be separated out from class, race and ethnicity, or age group. To give you an idea of some of the gendered patterns of morbidity and mortality that are the combined result of risky and protective behavior, environments, social expectations, and economic and other resources, I will organize them by life cycle—birth, adolescence and young adulthood, health behaviors in adulthood, work and family, old age, and death.

Birthing and Getting Born: Have Money or Be a Boy

For mothers, economic resources can spell the difference between life and death for their infants. In poor countries that favor men, all the advantages go to boys. The physical hazards that produce infertility are evenly incurred by men and women, but the social effects and treatments are much harder on women.

Childbirth and Infancy

One of the important contributors to women's longer life expectancy in the 20th century is the reduction of illness and death in childbirth.[3] The use of antibiotics for puerperal infections ("childbed fevers") and surgical interventions to prevent heavy blood loss has made dying in childbirth a rare occurrence in many countries. However, because of uneven access to prenatal care and safe abortions and inadequate treatment of childbirth complications, women in the childbearing years still suffer from high mortality and morbidity rates in many parts of the world, including the United States (Dixon-Mueller 1994; Sundari 1994). The health of the mother directly affects the health of the infant. In industrialized countries, the condition that enables us to predict with the greatest accuracy whether or not a baby will be stillborn, sick, malformed, premature, or will die in the first year of life, is the mother's socioeconomic status. If she belongs to a disadvantaged social class this means, among other things, low income, poor health, hard domestic and extra-domestic work, low educational level, and bad housing. (Romito and Hovelaque 1987:254)[4]

The more economic resources a country has, the better the health care and the lower the death rate of women in childbirth and their newborns in their first year.[5] Physiologically, girl babies are stronger at birth, and the female hormones generated at puberty are protective until menopause. However, women's longer life expectancy in developed countries, compared to men, reflects the effects of a healthier environment, better health care, and good nutrition, which are indicative of enough economic resources to feed women and girls as well as men and boys and to give pregnant women good health care (see Table 2.3). Another related set of statistics is whether or not girls and women are taught to read and write and the number of children they have. Educated women are good earners and too valuable to keep at home having children; hence, they have fewer and more widely spaced children and their maternal mortality rates drop.

In countries that put a high premium on having sons, neglect and infanticide of baby girls and deliberate abortions of female fetuses after prenatal sex testing has resulted in an imbalanced sex ratio (proportion of boys to girls or men to women) (Renteln 1992). Africa, Europe, and North America have a sex ratio of 95 girls to 100 boys, considered balanced because more boys than girls are born to compensate for the higher natural death rate of male children. In China, India, Bangladesh, and West Asia, the sex ratio is 94 girls to 100 boys, and in Pakistan it is 90 girls to 100 boys. Given the number of men, there should have been about 30 million more women in India today, and 38 million more women in China (Sen 1990).

These numbers do not necessarily reflect a complete devaluation of girls but rather a preference for boys if family size has to be limited. In China, for example, peasants feel that the ideal family is a son and a daughter; a daughter is an emotional and financial backup in case the son proves unfilial in the parents' old age (Greenhalgh and Li 1995). State policy, however, has forcefully discouraged a second child if the first is a son and forbidden a third child in almost all cases. Thus, many families have one or two sons and no daughters. Sex selection using amniocentesis occurs in the United States as well, but the practice is not well documented, and the effects have not significantly changed the ratio of girls to boys (Burke 1992).

Infertility

Although much of the research on fertility and birth focuses on women, it reflects the assumption that procreation is the concern of women because men can't get pregnant.[6] But men's fertility is just as vulnerable to environmental and occupational hazards as women's; toxic chemicals and other occupational hazards are equally likely to affect sperm production as viability of ova and fetal

Table 2.3

Health Care and Maternal and Infant Mortality Rates for Developed and Developing Countries

Region	% Prenatal Care 1990	% Attended by Trained Personnel	Maternal Mortality 1988[a]	Infant Mortality 1990-1995[a]
World	64	60	370	68
Developed	98	99	26	12
Developing	59	55	420	69
Africa	59	42	630	95
North America	95	99	12	8
Latin America[b]	72	76	200	47
Asia[c]	57	56	380	62
Europe	99	99	23	10
Former USSR	100	100	45	20
Oceania[d]	70	50	600	22

SOURCE: World Health Organization 1995:60.
a. Deaths per 100,000 live births.
b. Includes Mexico.
c. Excludes Japan.
d. Excludes Australia and New Zealand.

development (Bertin 1989; Hatch 1984; Vogel 1990).[7] Even with the knowledge of risk, there is little protection for workers in jobs where the workforce is predominantly women, such as nurses and anesthetists, who are exposed to radiation and powerful anesthetics, and assemblers in electronics factories, who work with potentially harmful solvents (Draper 1993). In 1991, the U.S. Supreme Court decided that employers could not use protection of the fetus as a rationale for barring fertile women from hazardous jobs. The decision to take a job that might cause infertility is now up to workers themselves (including men at risk of sperm deformity), but the government could insist that employers reduce *all* workers' exposure to occupational hazards or equip them with protective devices.[8]

Besides job-related hazards, sexually transmitted diseases, malnutrition, and inadequate health care have contributed to higher rates of infertility among African Americans, who are less likely to have access to expensive procreative technologies (Nsiah-Jefferson and Hall 1989). Recent data, however, indicate that their rates of both voluntary and involuntary childlessness are becoming similar to those of white Americans (Boyd 1989).

Infertility is more detrimental physiologically and socially for women than for men, even though male infertility has been very difficult to treat.[9] Women have more at stake but less bargaining power in the decisions over what to do about not being able to conceive. Whether the woman or the man is infertile, the woman is the one who usually seeks help. If she is determined to try to have a biological child with her partner, she has to assure his willingness to undergo whatever procedures physicians deem appropriate to their medical situation. She will also need his sympathy and emotional support throughout the days, months, and often years of repeated attempts to get pregnant. An infertile man might want to forget about having children entirely because he might feel that the examinations, tests, and intercourse and masturbation on demand sully his masculinity. Given his stress over his infertility, he might be unwilling or unable to provide much emotional support (Lorber and Bandlamudi 1993; Lorber and Greenfeld 1990; Nachtigall, Becker, and Wozny 1992).

The newest procreative technology, in vitro fertilization (IVF) or out-of-the-body conception, has been used in both female and male infertility. This method involves giving a woman hormones to make her produce more than one ovum a month, removing the ova, fertilizing them with sperm in a petri dish, and incubating the gametes for a day or two until the resultant cell division produces an embryo that can be implanted in the woman's womb (Fredericks, Paulson, and DeCherney 1987). In male infertility, IVF provides a technological means for a man who has low sperm count, poor sperm motility, or badly shaped sperm to impregnate and for his fertile partner to have *his* child (Spark 1988). In theory, IVF works in male infertility because a very small amount of good sperm is needed to get one to fertilize an egg in a petri dish. In the newest techniques, sperm is taken directly from the testicles, and just one is injected into an ovum (Palermo, Cohen, and Rosenwaks 1996). These procedures bypass common male infertility problems, but the success rate is quite low. In addition, the most difficult physical burdens are borne by the woman.

Most of the procedures, which involve not only administering hormones and surgery but many blood tests and sonograms, have to be undergone by the woman, who may be able to conceive with a much simpler procedure, donor insemination. If motherhood and not pregnancy is her goal, she may prefer to adopt. But if she refuses to undergo fertility treatments, her infertile male partner's opportunity to have a biological child in this relationship is lost. He has everything to gain and less to undergo. This imbalance in the demands of treatment sets up the dynamics of gender bargaining in male infertility (Lorber 1987, 1989; Lorber and Bandlamudi 1993). Some women also have procreative problems; others see the problem as theirs in any case. They are willing to undergo IVF when their male partner is infertile because they feel they have no other options to have a biological child. Some women who have no fertility problems do it for altruistic reasons, but some simply succumb to psychological pressure from their male partner.

Willingness to undergo repeated trials of IVF, even if they are unsuccessful, may be a rational decision for women, since families, the media, and the medical system all favor undergoing treatment.[10] Going through IVF proves to themselves, their mates, and family members that they have done everything they could to have a biological child together (Lorber and Greenfeld 1990). These latent gains are what make IVF so popular throughout the world, despite its low success rate of about 15 to 25 percent in female infertility and zero to 10 percent in male infertility. Doing IVF is often an obligatory rite of passage not only to try to have a child but also to try "to reach a secondary objective as a necessary substitute, that is, protection against social stigmatization and a means to obtain social recognition as an involuntary childless woman" (Koch 1990:240-41). Involuntary infertility is a form of sick role because the individual is not held responsible for her or his condition; to refuse treatment implies that the condition is voluntary and therefore not a true "illness" deserving sympathy and emotional support. Procreative pathology has its meaning within the social expectation that heterosexual adults have "their own" —biological—children if at all possible. Not being able to conceive does no harm physically but does so socially and psychologically; the treatment, however, can be physically as well as emotionally and financially costly, especially for women.

Adolescence and Young Adulthood: Good and Bad Social Pressures

Poor teenage girls in the United States are like women in poor countries—if they get good prenatal care and have social supports after the birth, they and their children thrive. But if they are stigmatized and therefore put off getting prenatal care, they are likely to have premature births and low-birth-weight babies, with accompanying health hazards. Even without childbirth, the lives of poor young men of color are the most endangered of all groups in the United States, exposing them to a host of physical and emotional traumas. Young women in college are prone to eating disorders, but in general, their health behaviors tend to be more protective than those of young men in college. The situation for young girls in non-Western countries, particularly in Africa, is starkly different. Genital mutilation is a gender-specific health issue in many countries of the world.[11]

Teenage Pregnancy

Teenage childbearing is a social problem that can be viewed from a health perspective (the effect on the body of a growing girl of having a baby in the teen years and the health of the infant) and from a social perspective (why teenage boys and girls want to have babies and what happens to those girls who do get pregnant). The data from recent research show that social conditions are more crucial than age or racial ethnic identity in predicting whether young, unmarried girls will have a pregnancy and what the physical and emotional outcome will be for the mother and the child (Luker 1996).

According to the providers in 200 randomly selected reproductive health and other service programs in New York City, girls of Puerto Rican and Dominican background got pregnant in their teen years because they lacked information about sexual relationships, procreation, and birth control (Fennelly 1993). But the reason why they couldn't acquire this knowledge was the contradictory attitudes of the Hispanic culture, attitudes that condemned sexuality outside of marriage but valued pregnancy and having children no matter when it occurred. The positive attitudes toward fatherhood among young men in many cultures and their intentions to play a significant role in the lives of their children and their children's mothers also make it difficult for teenage girls to practice birth control or have an abortion (Anderson 1989; Marsiglio 1988; Redmond 1985).

Once sexual activity begins, Black teenage girls from high-risk social environments are 8.3 times more likely to become pregnant than Black girls from low-risk social environments (Hogan and Kitagawa 1985). The data were based on a random sample of over 1,000 Black girls aged 13-19 who lived in Chicago in 1979. High risks in this study were being poor, living in an impoverished neighborhood with a non-nuclear family and many siblings, and having a sister who had also been a teenage mother. Another study interviewed 268 Canadian teenagers during pregnancy and four weeks after delivery and found that those who had strong support from their families were less likely to have low-birth-weight babies or postpartum depression (Turner, Grindstaff, and Phillips 1990).

Pregnancy soon after menarche is considered the norm in all but highly industrialized societies, and in most cultures, having a child, not marriage, is the mark of adulthood. In industrialized countries, the incidence of teenage pregnancy is low where sex education is part of the school curriculum and contraceptives and early abortions are widely available (Jones and Forrest 1985). Teenage pregnancy and childbirth may result in frequent premature births, which seems to be a more serious problem than low birthweight (Fraser 1995; Wilcox, Skjaerven, and Buekens 1995). Among Black women, premature births are high when there is a combination of related factors: teenage, single, no high school graduation, and welfare support (Lieberman et al. 1987). The major *social* (not physiological) problem for the teenage mother is the risk of ending up in poverty if she is not already poor or staying poor if she is (Chilman 1989; Forsyth and Palmer 1990; Luker 1996).

Endangered Species

Even with childbearing, young women are less vulnerable to early death than the young men of their racial ethnic groups. Because of multiple risk factors, young Black men living in disadvantaged environments are the most likely to die before they reach adulthood. Young Black men have been called an endangered species because of their early death rates, with homicides, suicides, and accidents the leading causes of death of those between 15 and 24 years old (Gibbs 1988; Staples 1995). For Black and white men between 15 and 19 years old, the annual homicide rate rose 154 percent from 1985 to 1991, with almost all of the increase due to the use of guns (Butterfield 1994). HIV infection and AIDS also have a high incidence in young Black and Hispanic men, especially when they are intravenous drug users. However, the consequent illnesses and deaths occur later, between the ages of 29 and 41 (Kranczer 1995).

Young men's "taste for risk" has been attributed to sociobiological factors (Wilson and Daly 1985), but more plausible explanations are the seductiveness of danger, displays of masculinity, and, for Black men, despair over the future

(Staples 1995). Another social factor is the recruitment into often violent sports (Messner 1992). Although a path to upward mobility for poor and working-class boys, few become successful professional athletes. Those who break into professional teams have only a few years to make it, and they cannot afford to be sidelined by injuries. "Playing hurt" and repeated orthopedic surgeries have a high physical toll. Injuries, alcoholism, drug abuse, obesity, and heart disease take about 15 years off the life expectancy of professional football players in the United States (Messner 1992:71).

Responses to Social Pressures

Health-threatening behavior, such as smoking, drinking, and illegal drug use, is influenced by a variety of social factors, but peer-group pressure is among the most significant for young men and women of all racial ethnic groups (Coombs, Paulson, and Richardson 1991; Johnson and Marcos 1988; Johnson 1988; van Roosmalen and McDaniel 1992). Drinking in college is declining among men and women, but college men still drink more often and more heavily than college women and are much more likely to get into fights, hurt others, drive while drunk, and damage property (Perkins 1992). Women as well as men who drink heavily are likely to hurt themselves physically and others emotionally and to do poorly in school.

Young women tend to adopt a somewhat healthier lifestyle than young men on such measures as using seat belts, getting adequate amounts of sleep and exercise, eating a healthy diet, taking care of their teeth, and managing stress (Donovan, Jessor and Costa 1993; Oleckno and Blacconiere 1990). However, young middle-class women are vulnerable to eating disorders, especially in the college years (Hesse-Biber 1989).

Anorexia (self-starvation) and bulimia (binge eating and induced vomiting) are extreme ways to lose weight in order to meet today's Western cultural standards of beauty and to maintain control over one's body (Bordo 1993; Brumberg 1988). The importance of society's views of femininity in eating disorders is highlighted by research comparing heterosexual women, who are subject to pressure from the media and the significant men in their lives to stay thin to be sexually attractive, and lesbians, whose views of beauty are not influenced by men's opinions. Lesbians are heavier than comparable heterosexual women, more satisfied with their bodies, and less likely to have eating disorders (Herzog et al. 1992). Men also have an idealized body image, which may encourage anorexia and bulimia, especially among those with sexual conflicts or who identify as homosexual (Herzog, Bradburn, and Newman 1990; Herzog et al. 1984; Kearney-Cooke and Steichen-Asch 1990).

A different rationale for eating problems was found in intensive interviews with 18 women who were heterogenous on race, class, and sexual orientation (Thompson 1992). For these African American, Latina, and white women, binge eating and purging were ways of coping with the traumas of their lives—sexual abuse, poverty, racism, and prejudice against lesbians. Eating offered the same comfort as drinking but was cheaper and more controllable. Rather than a response to the culture of thinness, anorexia and bulimia were for these women "serious responses to injustices" (Thompson 1992:558).

College athletes are prone to anorexia and bulimia when they have to diet to stay in a weight class (Andersen 1990; Black 1991). A study of 695 athletes in 15 college sports found that 1.6 percent of the men and 4.2 percent of the women met the American Psychiatric Association's criteria for anorexia, and 14.2 percent of the men and 39.2 percent of the women met the criteria for bulimia (Burckes-Miller and Black 1991). The researchers argue that the reasons for strict weight control are not standards of beauty but the pressures of competition, to meet weight category requirements, to increase speed and height, and to be able to be lifted and carried easily in performances. Eating disorders here are an occupational risk taken not only by young athletes but by dancers, models, jockeys, and fitness instructors as well as professional gymnasts, figure skaters, runners, swimmers, and wrestlers.

Genital Mutilation

For some young girls, being able to control the shape of your body by what you eat might look like paradise—not just to those who don't have enough to eat but to those girls aged 3 to 18 whose families insist on having their genitals amputated so that they can be properly married. Hanny Lightfoot-Klein (1989) estimated that 94 million women living in Africa in the 1980s had their clitorises and vaginal lips cut off (p. 31). In Egypt, an estimated 80-97 percent of girls have mutilated genitals (MacFarquhar 1996). These procedures are done on 90 percent of young girls in the Sudan and in Mali on 93 percent (Dugger 1996b). In 1996, the United States passed a law making all these procedures illegal, and other countries with large immigrant populations have also done so (Dugger 1996c).

For more than 2,000 years, in a broad belt across the middle of Africa, clitoridectomies and infibulation (scarring of the labia to create adhesions that keep most of the vaginal opening closed until marriage) have been used to ensure women's virginity until marriage and to inhibit wives' appetites for sexual relations after marriage. Ironically, these mutilating practices do neither but result in the infliction of pain as part of normal sexuality. Childbirth is more dangerous because of tearing and bleeding, and the risks of infection throughout life are high.

The procedures range from mild sunna (removing the prepuce of the clitoris) to modified sunna (partial or total clitoridectomy) to infibulation or pharaonic circumcision, which involves clitoridectomy and excision of the labia minora and the inner layers of the labia majora and suturing the raw edges together to form a bridge of scar tissue over the vaginal opening, leaving so small an opening that normal bladder emptying takes 15 minutes and menstrual blood backs up (see descriptions in Lightfoot-Klein 1989:32-36). Many women have reinfibulation after childbirth and go through the process over and over again. It is called *adlat el rujal* (men's circumcision) because it is designed to create greater sexual pleasure for men, not unlike the rationale for episiotomy and tight suturing in Western obstetrical practice (Rothman 1982:58-59).

In Lightfoot-Klein's (1989) interviews with women throughout the Sudan who had clitoridectomies and infibulation, 90 percent described experiencing full orgasms during intercourse once the period of excruciatingly painful opening through penile penetration was over. However, Asma El Dareer's (1982) survey of 2,375 women, almost all of whom had had full infibulation, found that only 25 percent experienced sexual pleasure all or some of the time (p. 48). One of the Sudanese men Lightfoot-Klein (1989) interviewed said that his wife's evident suffering was preferable to no reaction at all (p. 8).

Circumcision of boys is much more common and occurs in societies throughout the world, where it is done for both religious and health reasons. Although there is some debate over whether sensitivity is reduced or enhanced, male circumcision does not seem to diminish either the man's or the woman's pleasure (Gregersen 1983). Removal of the prepuce lowers the risk of HIV infection in circumcised men and cervical cancer in their women sexual partners. Another practice, subincision, where the penis is cut through and flattened and urination is subsequently done squatting, occurs in only a few places in the world.

Adulthood: Health by
Choice or by Circumstance?

Many of the risky health behaviors in adulthood, such as drinking and smoking cigarettes, seem to be a matter of individual choice. But a closer look reveals that social factors linked to gender, race and ethnicity, and economic class produce the situational circumstances that influence health-related behaviors.

A comparison of 654 African American and 474 white women aged 19 to over 70 living in upstate New York found that poorer, older, religious African American women were most likely to abstain from alcohol (Darrow et al. 1992). A study of 4,099 white women and men and 888 Black women and men living in New York State also found that Black women were most likely to abstain from drinking (Barr et al. 1993). Black men in this study were more likely than white men to abstain but also most likely, of all four groups, to be heavy drinkers when they did drink. A study of gendered styles of drinking showed that women of all racial ethnic groups who drank were less likely than men to become visibly intoxicated and to abandon control, behavior that would be considered un-feminine (Robbins and Martin 1993). When economic status was added to the analysis, it was found that the poorest and least educated Black men had significantly higher rates of alcohol and illicit drug consumption and alcohol-related problems, such as accidents and run-ins with the police, bosses, fellow workers, and family members. They are, as a result, more likely to suffer from high blood pressure and die early of coronary artery disease, especially if they also smoke (Staples 1995; Waldron 1995). The New York State study found that the more education a Black man had, the fewer alcohol-related problems he experienced, but that Black men with college degrees experienced such problems on an average of one a month, while their white counterparts averaged only 3.4

alcohol-related problems per year. Educated Black men are likely to be under increased stress because the stakes for success are so high.

Both legal and illegal drugs are commonly used by professional athletes (Messner 1992). Team doctors routinely inject painkillers and cortisone so injured players can "play hurt" and supply amphetamines to enhance performance and anabolic steroids to increase muscle mass. Steroid use among women and men bodybuilders who enter competitions is endemic, despite their virilizing effects in women and feminizing effects in men (Fussell 1993; Mansfield and McGinn 1993).

Among laypeople, women are more than twice as likely as men to be prescribed psychotropic drugs (tranquilizers and sleeping pills) for anxiety, but men often obtain such medications from women—their wives, sisters, or friends—when they are under stress because of their job or lack of one (Ettorre et al. 1994). Women and men physicians prescribe these medications to women more than they do to men with similar difficulties, but men physicians are significantly more likely to do so (Taggart et al. 1993). Elizabeth Ettorre and Elianne Riska (1995) argue that both the gendered use patterns and the prescribing patterns reflect powerlessness: Prescribing tranquilizers for women stressed out by their triple duties as wives, mothers, and paid workers treats the symptoms, not the causes, which women physicians are more likely to recognize. When men in difficult social situations ask sympathetic women they know rather than their men physicians for tranquilizers, the same gender dynamics of status and powerlessness seem to be at issue.

Homicide rates are greater for disadvantaged men but paradoxically, higher for educated women in the labor force (Gartner 1990). A cross-national, longitudinal comparison of 18 industrialized countries found that as women's lives between 1950 and 1985 moved away from traditional roles, they were more likely to be murdered (Gartner, Baker, and Pampel 1990). The researchers argue that, although women confined to the home are subject to violence from husbands and other men relatives, women who work for pay, especially in nontraditional occupations, and single women living on their own are also vulnerable to being killed by acquaintances and strangers.

The one place women maintain their life expectancy advantage despite risk behavior is with smoking—they outlive men even if they smoke heavily, leading to the conclusion that other factors provide protective health benefits for women (Rogers and Powell-Griner 1991).

Work and Family:
Protection and Danger

Jobs and families are complex variables with good and bad effects on the physical and mental health of women and men. Both are arenas for social support, which is beneficial to health; both are sometimes hazardous environments with detrimental physical effects; and both produce stresses.[12]

Work-Family Demands and Rewards

Although having a paid job outside the home usually enhances women's physical and mental health, jobs can be physically hazardous to women as well as men. Many of women's jobs are as physically dangerous as some men's jobs (Chavkin 1994; Fox 1991). Nursing, for example, can be highly stressful emotionally; hospitals also expose the nurse to infections, radiation, and dangerous chemicals (Coleman and Dickinson 1984; Kemp and Jenkins 1992). Full-time housewives are not protected either: The home is a similarly stressful and dangerous work environment full of toxic chemicals and potential allergens (Rosenberg 1984).

The job and the home can also produce high levels of psychological stress for women and men, and workplace and family stresses can spill over into each other (Eckenrode and Gore 1990). For women especially, the boundaries between work and family are permeable because even when they have full-time jobs they usually have the main responsibility for child care, household maintenance, and providing help to kin outside the household (Gerstel and Gallagher 1994; Lai 1995; Lennon and Rosenfeld 1992). In dual-career marriages, women often resent having a "double shift"—paid work plus housework—and men in turn feel that demands are made on them in the home that husbands in traditional marriages don't have (Glass and Fujimoto 1994). However, marriage extends men's and women's life spans but through different means, as suggested by Lillard and Waite (1995):

> "His" marriage seems to consist of a settled life, improved perhaps by the household management skills and labors of his wife. . . . "Her" marriage seems to offer primarily the benefits of improved financial well-being. (p. 1154)

The effects of workplace and family stress, role conflict, depression, and negative feelings on vulnerability to illness are hard to document. The connection between stress and heart attacks, for example, has not yet been proved (Waldron 1995). Moreover, some "hardy personalities" thrive under stress, according to a study of men executives (Maddi and Kobasa 1984; also see Ouellette 1993). A study of the effects of combined roles (work, marriage, and motherhood) in a sample of 1,473 Black and 1,301 white women found that work was significantly associated with lower blood pressure only for educated Black women (Orden et al. 1995). Being married was correlated with raised blood pressure for white women but with lower blood pressure during motherhood, even for single mothers. As an example of work's beneficial physical effects, separate studies found that older Black women and men had better health if they were employed (Coleman et al. 1987; Rushing, Ritter, and Burton 1992). This finding is not surprising, for employment usually means a higher income, which in turn means better nutrition and greater access to health care. Generally, people with health problems are not as able to hold down jobs as their healthier counterparts are.

The gender differences related to paid jobs and family demands are mini-mized when women and men live and work in similar unpressured environ-ments. A comparison of the health status of 230 women and men on two Israeli kibbutzes, where work and family life are communal and health care is free, found that they were alike in their health status and illness behavior and that the men had life expectancies as long as those of the women (Anson, Levenson, and Bonneh 1990).

Battering

The home is not only a place of potential environmental hazards and stress, it can also be the site of physical violence. The average yearly number of recorded acts of violence against women in the United States from 1979 to 1987 was 56,900 by husbands, 216,100 by divorced or separated husbands, and 198,800 by boy-friends (Harlow 1991:1).

Men whose masculinity is tied to norms of dominance but who do not have the economic status to back up a dominant stance are likely to be abusive to women either psychologically or physically and often both (Walker 1984; Yllö 1984). James Ptacek's (1988) interviews with 18 men in a counseling program for husbands who battered found that they felt they had a right to beat their wives:

> There is a pattern of finding fault with the woman for not being good at cooking, for not being sexually responsive, for not being deferential enough . . . , for not knowing when she is "supposed" to be silent, and for not being faithful. In short, for not being a "good wife." (p. 147)

Wife beating was once approved in most communities and is still condoned today where there is an ideology of men's authority over their wives. Marital rape has only recently been accorded recognition as a genuine sexual assault (Finkelhor and Yllö 1985). The response of doctors, nurses, and the police to battering reflects these mores. In general, neither the medical nor the legal system has given battered women much attention or protection (Blackman 1989; Kurz 1987; Warshaw 1989).

Women who stay in such relationships are likely to have been well socialized into the emotionally supportive feminine role but to be socially or economically superior to the men who batter them (Walker 1984). Beth Richie (1996) found that the 26 African American battered women she interviewed had had girlhoods of relative privilege and thought they could be ideal wives and mothers. They felt they could not admit to their families that they had failed to live up to their early promise as "good girls." They could not go to the police because their batterers had embroiled them in illegal activities. Julie Blackman's (1989) interviews with 172 battered women found that they did not have a sense of injustice over what was happening to them because they could not see any alternatives outside the situation. Even women who had acted on alternatives, such as calling the police or going to shelters for battered women, did not feel that they had severed the relationship.

Old Age: Women Live Longer But Not Better

Although the physiological aspects of old age seem to override social factors, in that women of every racial ethnic group in industrial societies outlive the men of their group, the quality of their lives in old age can suffer because of poverty and few social supports.

The later years of life present women and men with sex-specific health risks. The older men get, the more likely they are to develop prostate cancer, especially among Blacks (Weitz 1996). It can be cured by surgery, but the operation often has side effects, such as impotence and urinary incontinence. After menopause, women are faced with the question of whether to use estrogen replacement therapy, which carries the risk of breast cancer (Bush 1992). Without it, they may suffer from bone fragility and increased risk of heart disease (Bilezikian and Silverberg 1992; Jonas and Manolio 1996; Nachtigall and Nachtigall 1995).

In addition to these sex-specific physiological risks, social factors make getting older and dying different experiences for women and men. With longer life expectancy, many women in industrialized countries can expect to outlive their husbands or long-term male companions (Verbrugge 1989b). Most patients in places with Western medical systems go to a hospital for acute illnesses, surgery, and medical crises in chronic conditions, but hospitals in the United States now routinely send even very sick patients home within a week. Many more surgical procedures are done on an outpatient or one-night basis. With the shift of care from hospitals to home, someone needs to give medications and injections and change wound dressings (Glazer 1990). Even if home health care givers are hired, someone needs to supervise and fill in; this "someone" is usually a wife or other woman relative.

Shopping, cleaning, laundry, bedmaking, and paying bills are additional chores that women relatives do for sick and frail elderly persons living at home (Graham 1985). The question is, who takes care of elderly widows and those who have never married? Women 85 years and older are more likely than same-age men to be poor and living with relatives or in nursing homes (Longino 1988). Thus, for many women, the advantage of long life may not look like such a dividend after all.

Dying: Gendered Death Dips

One area in which social factors and physiological outcomes intertwine dramatically are "death dips." These are statistical drops in the expected rate of death in the weeks or days before a socially meaningful event followed by a statistical rise a week or two later. Since social meanings are gendered, one would expect that death dips would be, too—and so they are.

In his 1970 Princeton University doctoral dissertation, "Dying as a Form of Social Behavior," David P. Phillips documented an intriguing epidemiological statistic: that famous people were less likely to die in the month preceding their birthday than in the month after. He argued that they postponed death so as to participate in their public birthday celebrations. He also found, examining official tables of dates of death, that ordinary people postponed dying until after important social occasions, such as presidential elections in the United States, and among Jews, until after the holiest day of the year, the Day of Atonement (Yom Kippur), and Passover, the popular celebration of liberation from Egyptian slavery (Phillips and Feldman 1973; Phillips and King 1988).

This and subsequent research reveal that the death-dip phenomenon during major religious holidays is quite gendered because of the different meanings of these events for women and men (Idler and Kasl 1992; Phillips and King 1988; Phillips and Smith 1990; Reunanen 1993). The Passover death dip, for example, occurs only among men. There was a 25.8 percent rise in deaths in the week after Passover among white men with unambiguously Jewish names who died in California between 1966 and 1984; for women, there was no such difference in deaths immediately before and after Passover (Phillips and King 1988). Statistical analysis of the death rates in a different population found the same gender pattern for all the major Jewish holidays (Idler and Kasl 1992). These researchers' explanation is that Jewish men's involvement in religious observances is more central to their lives than it is to Jewish women, whose death patterns are similar to all nonobservant Jews: They are more likely to die in the month preceding a major holiday than in the month after, whereas Jewish men and all observant Jews are more likely to die in the month after (Idler and Kasl 1992:Table 4).[13]

The opposite pattern is true for Black and white Catholics and Protestants—women and men, observant and nonobservant, postpone death until after Christmas and Easter (Idler and Kasl 1992:Table 3). In fact, women are more likely to postpone dying until after these events, which tend to be family oriented rather than purely religious celebrations. A Finnish analysis of 60,000 deaths for the 1966-1986 period found that only women postponed dying until after Christmas, a family-centered holiday where the senior woman cooks the celebratory meal (Reunanen 1993).[14] A similar gendered phenomenon occurs around the Harvest Moon Festival among Chinese women aged 75 and older; their mortality rate is lower in the week before the holiday than in any other 6-month period studied (Phillips and Smith 1990). Older women play the central part in the Harvest Moon Festival; the senior woman of the household supervises daughters and daughters-in-law in the preparation of an elaborate meal. The shift in dying does not occur among elderly Chinese men.

The dip in expected deaths the week before a major religious festival and the concomitant rise the week after has been documented for Chinese women with cerebrovascular and cardiac diseases and for Jewish men with these diseases and also with malignant tumors (Phillips and Smith 1990). Such psychosomatic and gendered effects of social beliefs are even starker among Chinese Americans born in a year considered ill fated in Chinese astrology who have a disease considered particularly detrimental for that birth year (Phillips, Ruth, and Wagner 1993).

Their average age of death occurs almost two years earlier than among non-Chinese and those born in more advantageous years who have the same illnesses. Women with the ill-fated combination of birth year and disease lose more years of life than men. The gender pattern, Phillips et al. (1993) speculate, is due to greater traditionalism among Chinese American women. However, the researchers argue that the crucial factors involve behavior as well as beliefs:

> Patients with ill-fated combinations of birth year and disease may refuse to change unhealthy habits because they believe their deaths are inevitable and thereby reduce their longevity. For example, earth patients with cancer may be less likely to quit smoking and fire patients with heart disease may be less likely to change their diets or exercise habits. (p. 1144)

How should a social epidemiologist classify these early deaths? Is the cause individual behavior, cultural beliefs, community practices, gender, race, or social class? Or all the above?

Summary

Basic epidemiological statistics, such as life expectancy, cause of death, and illnesses throughout life, reflect the economic resources of a society and the social status of women and men and girls and boys.

Women's longer life expectancy in modern industrialized societies depends in great part on access to medical care in pregnancy and childbirth. The effects of childbearing in adolescence, which often results in premature births and low-birth-weight infants who may be physically underdeveloped, are outcomes of poverty, lack of prenatal care, and few social supports. When friends and family provide care and concern during pregnancies, the outcome is likely to be physically and psychologically favorable for both infants and mothers.

Hazardous work environments affect fetal development and sperm production and may result in infertility in men as well as women. In both social stigma and extensiveness of treatment, however, the burden of infertility is much greater for women than for men.

The available data on Black and Hispanic adolescents of both genders indicate that all are more vulnerable to poor health and early death because they live in dangerous social environments, but that girls and young women are less likely than boys and young men to engage in health-endangering behavior. Because of the combination of social factors in their disadvantaged neighborhoods and in their compensatory risk-defying actions, young Black and Hispanic men in United States inner cities have high rates of death from homicide, suicide, and accidents before they reach adulthood and from AIDS later on. A social practice with severely detrimental physical effects is mutilation of the genitals of young girls to keep them chaste and marriageable. This practice is very widespread in Egypt and throughout Africa.

In adulthood, economic factors affect the health risks of women and men of various racial ethnic groups differently: Economically disadvantaged men are more vulnerable to occupational traumas and homicide and women to having and raising children in poverty. For all adults, smoking, drinking, taking drugs, lack of exercise, and poor diets are health-related behaviors somewhat under individual control, although having the time to exercise and the money to buy nutritional food may be large situational obstacles to a healthy lifestyle. Peer-group and family supports—social, psychological, and economic—influence individual health behaviors. These supports can be detrimental as well as protective, and their effects are gendered. For instance, peer groups encourage alcohol consumption among college men and extreme forms of dieting among college women. But eating and drinking problems can also be responses to poverty and prejudice.

Juggling work and family responsibility may be more stressful for women than for men, but employment is beneficial to the physical and mental health of both women and men, providing not only income but a social circle. Having little control over one's work situation produces a high level of stress, so that people in low-level jobs and middle management may suffer more depression and psychosomatic illnesses than those in high positions. Men from disadvantaged racial ethnic groups and all women are most likely to have jobs with little mobility and autonomy. However, stress may not always be detrimental to health; some people have been found to thrive on it.

The home can also be the site of violence: Most women who are battered suffer at the hands of their husbands and lovers. A few fight back, and when they do, the violence escalates, often ending in homicide (Walker 1989).

Old age and dying, like being born, is a gendered social phenomenon. Life expectancy and timing of death are influenced as much by social as physiological factors. Religion, family, income, and access to medical care are significant in the longevity and quality of life of elderly women and men.

The "death dip" phenomena, in which people with chronic or terminal illnesses postpone dying until after a meaningful event, such as a birthday, national election, or religious holiday, demonstrate the power of the social and psychological over physiology. The influence of gender is evident in the variable meaning of these events to different groups of women and men.

In sum, throughout life the human experiences of birth, death, disability, and illness are embedded in social contexts. Because gender is such an important part of social life, women's and men's experiences are different in sickness and in health, when rich and when poor, and in death, quite far apart.

Notes

1. On the problems of constructing categories of race and ethnicity, see Jones, Snider, and Warren 1996.

2. A substantial proportion of some morbidity rates are not explained by well-known risk factors. In breast cancer, for instance, only half of the cases in the United States are related to early menarche, having a family history of breast cancer or a personal history of benign breast disease, having a baby after

the age of 19 or not having children, and being in the upper two-thirds in income (Madigan et al. 1995). Note that these factors are both physiological and social and that the social factors are circumstances over which a woman may have little control. Breast cancer genes account for only 10% of all breast cancer cases (Biesecker and Brody, 1997).

3. For the detrimental effects of extensive technology in childbirth, see Rothman 1982, 1986, 1989.

4. In her editorial preface to the September/October 1995 issue of the *Journal of the American Medical Women's Association,* which is devoted to prenatal care and women's health, Wendy Chavkin notes that "the common thread woven throughout these articles is that improvements in pregnancy outcome require care for women before and after pregnancy" (p. 143). See also Lazarus 1988a and Lieberman et al. 1987.

5. For a detailed and harrowing account of how mothers in the poorest area of Brazil choose which of their infants to feed and which to let die, see Scheper-Hughes 1992.

6. Theoretically, it is physiologically possible for a man to gestate a fetus (Teresi 1994).

7. According to a review of studies of dropping sperm counts and sperm quality in Western countries, men's fertility may be on the endangered list (Wright 1996).

8. For discussions of the political and policy issues, see Merrick and Blank 1993.

9. Abbey, Andrews, and Halman 1991; Andrews, Abbey, and Halman 1991; Greil 1991; Lasker and Borg 1995; Miall 1986; Pfeffer 1987; Sandelowski 1993; and Spark 1988.

10. Callan et al. 1988; Crowe 1985; Franklin 1990; Koch 1990; and Williams 1988.

11. Immigration and asylum seekers have brought genital mutilation to the attention of Western countries (see Crossette 1995; Dugger 1996a, 1996b, 1996c; MacFarquhar 1996; Rosenthal 1996; Walker 1992).

12. For reviews and research, see Bird and Fremont 1991; Farrell and Markides 1985; Gove 1984; Lennon 1994; Loscosso and Spitze 1990; Muller 1990; Pugliesi 1995; Roxburgh 1996; Sorensen and Verbrugge 1987; and Waldron 1995.

13. Idler and Kasl did not break down their observant versus nonobservant data by gender.

14. I am indebted to Elianne Riska for bringing this paper to my attention and for supplying me with an English summary and a description of Finnish Christmas customs.

CHAPTER 3

The Doctor Knows Best

Gender and the Medical Encounter

I really don't know whether the influx of Blacks and women will change
the medical profession in any fundamental way. The way medical
education is, I think that sometimes there's a role that they want you to
fill, and the pressures to conform to that role are so strong. There's a
whole thing that if you're different, you're ostracized, you feel that you
don't know as much. There have been some changes, but I don't know
how widespread they're going to be. (Gamble 1982:258)

In Chapter 2, I described the kinds and rates of illnesses that differ by gender as
well as by social class and race. These mortality and morbidity statistics are
predominantly the results of social and economic advantages and disadvantages,
access to medical resources, family support or neglect, gendered lifestyles, and
individual behaviors and attitudes. The subject of this chapter is how people with
those illnesses are treated in Western medicine. "Western medicine" is the term
used for a system of health care whose knowledge base is modern science and
whose practitioners are licensed by the government of the country in which they
practice (in the United States, the state). The licenses (M.D., R.N., D.D.S., and so
on) are issued after the candidate has learned a standardized curriculum and
passed a standardized test. The curriculum, teaching, and testing are under the
control of the current holders of the license; in other words, professional qualifica-
tions are controlled by the respective profession. Each holder of a "doctor" license
is equal to any other doctor; nurses, however, have to obey doctors' orders. In all
the countries with Western medical systems, most of the nurses are women; in
many countries, most of the physicians are men. Although more and more
women are going into medicine and men into nursing, the gendered hierarchy
built into the structure of the two major and complementary health care professions in Western medicine has not been completely eroded. In this hierarchy,
medicine is the privileged profession—with greater authority and prestige and
higher income. The one exception was the former Soviet Union: In the state
medical system, women physicians predominated, but they were not highly paid
and did not have high status; their social standing was similar to women teachers
in the United States (Lorber 1984:26-27).

Most sick people throughout the world are not treated in a Westernized medical system. In the past, most illnesses were treated by family members or by healers who lived in the community or traveled through neighboring towns. Their medicines were herbal or animal based; their techniques relied on skilled hands; their education was through an apprenticeship with an experienced bonesetter, tooth puller, leecher, bloodletter, cupper, trepanner, military surgeon, or midwife.[1] Every racial-ethnic group has had a native medicine, with men and women healers. To this day, people of every social class in every country of the world consult native healers or use alternative medical treatments, even when they use "official," or Western, medicine (Kessler et al. 1993; Kolata 1996; Morgan 1983; Wilkinson and Sussman 1987).[2] In countries like India and China, native medicine is a recognized parallel system, with its own medical schools, hospitals, and clinics (*Barefoot Doctor's Manual* 1977; Leslie 1976). In the United States, 10 states license naturopathic doctors, who use diet, exercise, vitamins, herbal remedies, massage, meditation, and acupuncture (Egan 1996). In 1992, the National Institutes of Health set up the Office of Alternative Medicine, which supports evaluation research on these treatments. HMOs have used relaxation and meditation techniques, and even prayer, and in Seattle, voters have approved the establishment of a government-supported natural medicine clinic (Egan 1996; Hilts 1995). Because alternative medicine is not "scientific," some doctors deplore its legitimation (Park and Goodenough 1996).

The first Western medical schools were set up in medieval and early modern Europe in church-run universities. The curriculum, taken from the writings of the famous Greek physicians, Hippocrates and Galen, and Islamic medicine, was taught in Latin, and doctors still write prescriptions and many medical orders in Latin. Although at the time there were educated women physicians, whose writings were well known, women were excluded from the faculty and student body of the church-run universities (Green 1989; Siraisi 1990:27) and their writings were not used in the curriculum. University-educated doctors worked only for the nobility or gentry, so women practitioners and non-university-trained men had plenty of patients, many of whom consulted their written treatises on medicine.

The university-trained doctors did not have a better cure rate. Like all practitioners at the time, to make a diagnosis they relied on their five senses (sight, touch, hearing, smell, and taste) and patients' description of symptoms and then attempted a cure using bloodletting and purging techniques.[3] Fortunately for patients' survival, most illnesses are self-limited, and the placebo effect, or power of suggestion, also enhances the cure rate. The division of doctors into university-trained and lay healers was a class distinction, not one of knowledge or theory. If anything, lay healers probably had a higher cure rate because they had more hands-on experience and used medications that had worked for them in the past.

Most of the major discoveries that moved Western medicine beyond Greco-Islamic texts and localized knowledge did not come from university-trained doctors but from European amateur scientists, commercial chemists, and public health officers who worked in the 18th and 19th centuries. Leeuwenhoek, a Dutch lens maker, built a microscope and saw his own sperm move. Jenner, a British public health officer, noting that milkmaids did not get smallpox but the milder cowpox, developed the first vaccine. Pasteur, a French chemist trying to prevent wine from turning to vinegar and milk from going sour, theorized that something similar in both was producing the chemical changes. It took another generation for this seemingly disparate information to come together in the theory that the bacteria (then called "germs") in water, milk, wine, blood, and pus were the underlying cause of many diseases.

Semmelweis, an Austrian physician who headed a big lying-in hospital in Vienna, couldn't figure out why the rate of childbirth fever was so much higher in the wards run by physicians and medical students compared to those run by midwives until he realized that the doctors and students did autopsies on women who had died of the fever, and the midwives did not. He instituted the highly unusual practice of making the staff wash their hands in an antiseptic before they delivered or examined a woman internally, and the fever rate plummeted. He knew that something was carried in blood and pus, but because the germ theory of disease had not been formulated or disseminated among practicing physicians, he was considered a crackpot. When he left, the situation went back to the status quo, and he died insane.

Although the women involved in these and other famous discoveries were very aware of what was going on—birthing women in Semmelweis's hospital fought to go to the midwives' wards—their observations were not written down. Their knowledge was co-opted and monopolized by the men who wrote up their discoveries for publication; the women's contributions were subsumed in the knowledge base the men developed for the new medical science (Foucault 1975).

Gender and Physician Dominance

Licensed physicians' superior position in the United States occurred in the early part of the 20th century, when American physicians who had been trained in European medical schools recommended replacing the apprenticeship and six-week course of lectures that had been the standard in the 19th century with two years of science and two years of bedside learning. Only graduates of the reformed medical schools would receive the M.D. degree and be licensed to practice medicine. The combination of these two reforms produced a revolutionary transformation.[4] The adoption of the enhanced curriculum meant that many medical schools closed and fewer physicians were trained. Medicine became an elite profession that systematically excluded or set quotas for all women and African American, Jewish, and Catholic men (Moldow 1987; Starr 1982; Walsh 1977).[5] Medical practice became oriented to science and disease, neglecting prevention and environmental and social concerns. Doctors trusted only what they had learned in medical school and their own clinical experience and discounted nurses', midwives', and patients' knowledge.

Physicians' dominant position in Western medicine was bolstered by new medicines such as insulin for diabetes and penicillin and other antibiotics for infections. Their effectiveness in treating common illnesses eventually helped convince the skeptical that they were better off consulting an expensive physician than dosing themselves with home remedies or getting care from familiar community-based practitioners, such as midwives, homeopaths, and native medicine healers. What made physicians the final authority and gatekeeper to services within Western medical systems was state enforcement—only licensed M.D.s are allowed to prescribe many drugs and do most surgical procedures. Other licensed medical practitioners, such as midwives, physicians' assistants, and nurse practitioners, may work independently, but they are limited in what they can do.[6] This hierarchy of authority does not always derive from having more or less expert knowledge; doctors overrule nurses even when nurses know more about a case.

The fight for turf in the medical system is ongoing, and gender has been a weapon used by both women and men. In the battle to upgrade the profession of medicine in the United States, women physicians insisted that they were better doctors for women and children because of their life experiences; their men competitors claimed superior scientific knowledge, which they monopolized by keeping women students out of the reformed medical schools (Morantz-Sanchez 1985; Walsh 1977). In actuality, the clinics and hospitals run by women physicians in the late 19th century took care of women patients' social needs *and* had a lower infection rate than most facilities run by men physicians (Drachman 1984).

Today, women enter medical schools in many countries in large numbers, but they still encounter sexism. They are still encouraged to go into the classic women's specialties—pediatrics and family medicine—or into one of today's growing fields for women—obstetrics and gynecology, ophthalmology, and dermatology. Neurology, surgery, cardiology, and orthopedics, which are higher-paid, more prestigious specialties, are still men's provinces. The top positions of large medical centers, medical schools, and research centers are rarely held by women.[7] These institutions are where medical knowledge is developed, and so, for many patients, the authoritative voice of the physician continues to be a man's.

Nurses: Doctors' Handmaidens or Partners?[8]

Before the late 19th century, women nurses traditionally were either nuns or women down on their luck. Florence Nightingale chose middle- and upper-class "gentlewomen" for her nursing schools but made them handmaidens to men physicians by forbidding them to do anything—even giving a patient a drink of water—without a doctor's order. She did this because she wanted nursing to be *medical* work rather than something that women did as wives, mothers, nuns, or servants. She succeeded in upgrading and professionalizing nursing through a curriculum that combined basic medical science with hygiene and hands-on bedside care. Everything the nurse did was to be medically therapeutic. When hospitalized patients' emotions and social situations were discovered in the mid-20th century to have an impact on their recovery rates, TLC (tender loving care) was added to nursing practice. In theory, the nurse was to be "mother" to the physician "father," equally responsible for the patient "child." In practice, however, the nurses' job is documenting and carrying out physicians' orders for medication and hooking up and watching machines (Strauss et al. 1985). If patients get any attention to their emotional needs in hospital settings, it is from women at the bottom of the hierarchy, such as nurses' aides and nursing home attendants, who are ironically paid only for physical care (Diamond 1986).

The nursing profession's own hierarchy (nurses with college education vs. practical nurses) is racially stratified (Butter et al. 1987; Glazer 1991; Glenn 1992). Men nurses (about 6 percent in the United States) tend to gravitate to administration, an interesting example of the gender effects of tokenism. Christine Williams (1989, 1992, 1995) found that men nurses in the United States are tracked into the more prestigious, better-paying specialties within nursing and urged by their mentors to move into positions of authority.[9] Not to move up to supervisory and administrative positions is considered inappropriate. As a result, they are on a "glass escalator," upwardly mobile whether they are ambitious or not (Williams 1992), but they sometimes face the "glass ceiling" at higher levels. The affirmative action policies of many institutions make the women heads of nursing too visible for them to be replaced by men.

Although nurses are all formally subordinates of physicians, men and women nurses have different informal relationships with men and women physicians. Men nurses can talk about sports and other masculine subjects with men physicians (Williams 1989:118-19). They may gain a benefit from these informal contacts in more favorable evaluations of their work. Men physicians' status is too high to be compromised by chatting with men nurses (or bantering with women nurses). In hospitals, women physicians socialize with women medical students, interns, and residents but rarely with women nurses (Lorber 1984:60-61). They need to get along with the women nurses so that their work proceeds efficiently, but they lose status if they bond with lower-status women.

Whether they are men or women, administrators or bedside caretakers, nurses' structural position in the Western medical care system is subordinate to physicians when they work as a team because the holder of the M.D. has the ultimate authority over and responsibility for patients' treatment (Freidson 1970b). Nurse practitioners and nurse midwives work independently, but they cannot write prescriptions or admit patients to hospitals and usually are not reimbursed directly by insurance companies. Nurses' training and practice is in *care*, which "blurs the distinction between the medical and the social, the physiological and the psychological" (Fisher 1995:10), but their influence is constrained by their subordinate structural position. Unlike medicine, in which all holders of M.D. degrees are professional equals, nursing is stratified by education and type of degree—registered nurses (RNs) have two or more years of college and licensed practical nurses (LPNs) have only nursing school training. In the United States, the nursing hierarchy is racially and ethnically segregated, with the lower ranks predominantly African American and Hispanic (Glazer 1991, Glenn 1992, Hine 1989).

Thus, although the majority of the professional health care workers in Western medicine are women, the power and prestige (and high income) accrue to men because they predominate in policy-making positions and in the better-paid specialties. The health-care pyramid has women practical nurses and nursing-home attendants at the base, with mostly women registered nurses and women midwives one level higher. Further up the hierarchy are nurse supervisors and administrators and office-based primary care physicians (predominantly women). At the top are heads of large medical centers, chiefs of hospital and medical school departments, and prestigious specialists (predominantly men). It is within this gendered structure that laypeople encounter medicine.

The Medical Encounter

When patients go to see doctors, physicians ask the questions and patients give the answers. However, not all patients' answers are listened to. In fact, sometimes their voice is not heard at all; only their body is allowed to "speak":

> It happened the other morning on rounds, as it often does, that while I was carefully auscultating a patient's chest, he began to ask me a question. "Quiet," I said, "I can't hear you while I'm listening." (Baron 1985:606)

Doctors listen for *symptoms*—medical evidence of what the patient could be sick with or signposts of the progress of an already diagnosed disorder. They discount much of the patient's narrative of how this illness episode came about as irrelevant, even though it usually explains the circumstances under which the symptoms arose or got worse. The physician's perspective is the "voice of medicine"; the patient talks with the "voice of the lifeworld." These voices represent "the technical-scientific assumptions of medicine and the natural attitude of everyday life" (Mishler 1984:14). Both voices need to be heard to understand an illness in its entirety, but, except for those physicians consciously practicing holistic medicine, the voice of medicine usually prevails over the lifeworld voice.

The reason is that doctors are trained in the biomedical model, which locates illness in the body, not the social environment (Good and Good 1993; Mishler 1981). They are also trained to look for specific causes for illnesses and to rely on the scientific and technological tools of their trade—stethoscopes, X rays and CAT scans, blood counts, and other laboratory tests of bodily fluids and specimens (Reiser 1978). Although patients' accounts of their illnesses could provide valuable supplemental data to these objective findings, physicians tend to discount them as *subjective* and therefore unreliable. In actuality, the technological data have a heavy input of subjectivity, too, since what is heard through a stethoscope, counted in a complete blood workup, and seen on X-ray films and sonogram screens has to be interpreted—the "facts" never "speak for themselves" (Atkinson 1995; Lindenbaum and Lock 1993; Wright and Treacher 1982).

Physicians' interpretations, however, are seen as value neutral, carrying the weight of universal scientific fact:

> The medical encounter is one arena where the dominant ideologies of society are promulgated and where individuals' acquiescence is sought. The subtle force of this phenomenon derives from the presumed objectivity and helpfulness that the symbolism of scientific medicine conveys. (Waitzkin 1983:181)[10]

Comparisons of physicians' decisions based on similar symptoms and test results, however, show significant variation linked to the doctors' professional status and practice settings and their and the patients' social characteristics, especially gender.

Regardless of the extent of any individual physician's knowledge, expertise, or biases, the medical system legitimizes the holder of the M.D. as the official authority and downgrades what the patient or any other health care worker knows or thinks (Davis 1988). Patients able to pay for many visits can "doctor shop" to find a physician who will order the services they want, and they also use alternative medical practitioners at the same time as M.D.s. These are forms of resistance that do not change the system itself. Similarly, supplemental care by midwives, nurses, and physicians' assistants may offer patients more "user friendly" services but does not alter the medical hierarchy (Lazarus 1988b, 1990, 1994; Rothman 1982).

Doctors' power and authority in the medical encounter derive from their gatekeeping position in the social structure of Western medicine. Doctors are mandated by law and by the policies of health care agencies to validate whether or not someone is sick enough to get services, and they also determine which of the available (or insured) services a patient will get. Patients can circumvent their physicians by going to alternative healers or by paying for the services of other health professionals. They can also bargain with their physicians for the services they think they need. The theoretical context for the doctor-patient relationship is a central concept in medical sociology—the *sick role.*

The Gendered Sick Role[11]

The sociological dimensions of the sick role were first described by Talcott Parsons (1951). Parsons compared illness and crime as forms of deviance and the medical and legal systems as agents of social control. He argued that criminals and ill persons were deviant because they did not participate in normal roles— especially work roles. Unlike criminals, ill persons could not be held responsible for their condition and therefore could not be punished for being unable to fulfill normal social obligations. Ill persons were, however, held responsible for recognizing that the problem was beyond their ability to handle, for seeking competent professional help, and for wanting to get well. (The components of the sick role are shown in Figure 3.1.)

Working with "ideal types," Parson's model of the sick role assumed voluntary action on the part of the person with symptoms, a consensus of values and

Norms for Person With Symptoms	Norms for Family and Friends
No-Fault Incapacity Patient is not blamed for inability to go to work or school or for not meeting other normal social obligations.	*Permissiveness* Others should give support, sympathy, concern, care.
Conditional Deviance If condition persists, the social systems the individual is involved in (work, family) will be disrupted; therefore, to legitimate continued exemption from social responsibilities, the individual must recognize that the condition is beyond his or her capacity to handle and must seek professional help.	*Lay Referral* Ill person consults with family and friends over possible reasons for the symptoms (lay diagnoses), what kind of professional help is needed, and who should be consulted for that help.

Norms For Patients	Norms For Health Personnel
Help Seeking Help must be sought only in the medical system recognized in the community and with legitimate and appropriate health care personnel.	*Search for Diagnosis and Treatment* While a diagnosis is being made and appropriate treatment prescribed, patient is given permission to continue exemption from normal social obligations. Bed rest or hospitalization may be imposed.
Cooperation Patient must put self in hands of professional, accept diagnosis, and follow prescribed treatment regimen.	*Manipulation of Rewards* Professional must not foster long-term dependency but encourage patient to want to get well.
Return to Normalcy Goal is restoration to normal social roles or management of daily living to be as close to normal as possible.	*Social Control* Professional is an advocate of society as well as of the patient—must restore "order" by returning patient to normal roles or designating patient permanently disabled.

Figure 3.1 *The Sick Role*

goals for laypeople and health care personnel, and an always helpful professional. For him, the medical encounter was good for society as well as for the patient. Patients benefited by expert help for a problem beyond their competence to handle and by a return to normal functioning. Society benefited by physicians' documentation of "true illness" so that malingerers and hypochondriacs could not use medical resources or receive government support. What Parsons did not see was that physicians acting as society's agents in the determination of medical needs could be detrimental to patients' well-being, as when doctors in training recommend hysterectomies for poor women in order to get surgical experience, and then, when their techniques have been perfected, operate only on those patients who can pay them (Scully [1980] 1994).

In *Profession of Medicine*, Eliot Freidson (1970a) described the conflicts in the sick role and the negative effects of becoming a patient. Men may deny their inability to carry out normal obligations because they have been taught to be stoical; women become patients when they see a doctor for contraceptive or other gynecological services. Low-paid women and men workers may have to continue to work despite pain or fever because they have no sick leave or health insurance. Family members may not be supportive of women homemakers' laying down on the job. Patients and physicians may disagree over diagnoses or treatments, but hospitalized patients learn to keep quiet and do what they are told; the lower their social status, the more likely they are to follow "good patient" norms (Lorber 1975b). Battered women find that when they seek emergency care the social circumstances of their traumas are ignored and only their wounds and broken bones are treated (Kurz 1987; Warshaw 1989, 1996). Patients may benefit when alcoholism or drug use are considered illnesses rather than crimes or sins but still be stigmatized even if the illness is cured. A return to normal social status in any illness may be foreclosed by the possibility of relapse or recurrence and lack of caretakers. The physician's goal is to return patients to normal functioning, and for many physicians that means a job for a man and homemaking and child care for a woman (Waitzkin 1991).

The medical encounter, in short, may not be so benign: Doctors may not always look out for patients' best interests; patients' social circumstances may be ignored and their marital and sexual status stereotyped; and the diagnosis or treatment may be stigmatizing. Yet they have to seek doctors' help because the physician in Western medicine is the official expert and also the ultimate gate-keeper to most of the services a patient needs, such as prescription medicines, diagnostic tests, and hospital care.

To obtain the privilege of exemption from normal social obligations in countries with Westernized medical systems, you must enter the health care system and be documented as legitimately ill—we call it getting a "doctor's note." If the doctor or the doctor's surrogate does not validate the illness, you are not likely to get extended sick leave days from your workplace or makeup tests from your teachers. Without official legitimation, anyone could claim the privilege of not working or not going to school and being cared for by others with the simple declaration that he or she was sick. A physician's documentation is needed to become an official patient, to get most medical services, insurance reimbursement, and hospital care, to be legally disabled, and even to be officially born or dead.

These legal requirements to see a physician keep sick people under the control of the medical system, which, as has been seen, is stratified and segregated by gender, race, and social class. As it affects the doctor-patient relationship, gender stratification means that men doctors are more likely to be specialists and women doctors to be in primary care. The physician's gender and race, specialty, practice setting (office, outpatient clinic, hospital), and age combine with the patient's gender, race, and age to produce outcomes that have significant effects on how the medical encounter proceeds.

Gender and Medical Practice[12]

According to recent data on medical practice, gender makes a difference in two ways: Women and men patients are treated differently, and women and men physicians treat women patients differently. In the United States, women patients with symptoms of heart disease are treated less aggressively than men patients, and women physicians are more likely than men physicians to order Pap tests and mammograms for their women patients.

Even though coronary heart disease is the major cause of death in the United States, women are less likely than men to be routinely tested for cardiovascular symptoms and more likely to suffer unrecognized heart attacks (Hendel and Mendelson 1995; McKinlay 1996; Wingard et al. 1992). Women who come to the doctor with severe symptoms are not as likely as men with lesser symptoms to be given a coronary arteriography, catheterization, or bypass surgery (Steingart et al. 1991; Wenger 1994). As a result, they are more likely than men of the same age to die if they have a myocardial infarction, and the postoperative mortality rate for coronary artery bypass surgery has been found to be significantly higher in women than in men (Hsia 1993). When women do have coronary artery bypass surgery, they are more likely to be given sedatives for anxiety and agitation rather than narcotic analgesics for postoperative pain (Calderone 1990).

One woman physician argued that the blame cannot be placed only on physicians' shoulders for the minimization of women's cardiovascular risk; the woman herself and her family and friends also need to be made aware that as women get older they are at as great a risk as middle-aged men from the long-term effects of coronary artery problems:

> Unless society perceives of coronary disease as an important illness in older
> women, the older woman recommended for diagnostic testing for chest pain
> is less likely to receive reinforcement to do so from family and friends, as is
> the case when such testing is recommended for men. (Wenger 1994:185)

However, it is the physician's authority and expertise that influence what laypeople think, and here the patient's gender makes a significant difference. Too many physicians still act as if only men had heart attacks (American Medical Association Council 1991).

In an area of medical practice where the risks for women are well known— breast and cervical cancer—as are the guidelines for regular Pap smears and mammograms, whether they are recommended seems to depend on the gender of the physician. Studies covering thousands of patients in the United States have found large, statistically significant differences between the recommendations for these tests by women and men physicians. In one study of a national sample of 5,536 women, the more than 90 percent with men health care providers were less likely than those with women physicians to have had a Pap test in the previous three years and for those over 45 to ever have had a mammogram (Franks and Clancy 1993).

Another study, which used the records of a large midwestern medical health plan, found that women who were patients of women doctors were nearly twice as likely to have received a Pap test and 40 percent more likely to have had a mammogram the previous year than women who had seen men doctors (Lurie et al. 1993). The researchers analyzed the claims for Pap smears and mammographies of 27,713 women patients who had seen only one physician the previous year for the gender, age, and specialty of that doctor. They found that 550 physicians were in internal medicine and family practice and another 130 in obstetrics-gynecology. Twenty percent of all these physicians were women, and they were about 10 years younger than the men physicians. Among the gynecologists, the younger men physicians (38 to 42 years old) were less likely than all the women and the older men to order cancer-screening tests. Among the internists and family practitioners, the men physicians ordered significantly fewer of these tests than the women physicians, with those under 38 years of age having the lowest rates of all. The authors of this study questioned why, among younger physicians, whose medical education has stressed the need for preventive screening, men are so reluctant to recommend Pap smears and mammograms to their women patients. They posited that perhaps these tests were easier to discuss when the doctor and patient were of the same gender. However, such reluctance in men gynecologists is surprising.

A study that focused on family practitioners added cholesterol testing—a gender-neutral area (Kreuter et al. 1995). The researchers interviewed women patients in 12 family practices in North Carolina—1,630 whose regular provider was 1 of 33 men physicians, and 220 who usually saw 1 of 5 women physicians—and found that among patients older than 20 who had not had a cholesterol test in five years, those seeing a woman doctor were 56 percent more likely to get the test than those seeing a man doctor.

In short, women patients, who make more visits to physicians, do not get the best treatment for heart disease nor do they get good preventive care, even in well-known, high-risk breast and cervical cancers, unless they have a woman doctor. Their longer life expectancy cannot be attributed to medicine but is much more likely the result of engaging less in risky behavior, such as smoking. But since vulnerability to breast cancer is a combination of genetic and environmental factors, such as place of residence, and cervical cancer rates are affected by the behavior and health status of male partners, women have to rely on early detection for protection—and that means reliance on a gender-biased medical profession (Fisher 1986).[13]

Do Women Physicians Have
More Caring Practice Styles?

Today, men and women physicians acknowledge the necessity to understand their patients' daily lives, work and family roles, and emotional needs when they are treating them for a physical illness, but patients claim that women doctors are more "humane" (Fennema, Meyer, and Owen 1990). Women physicians may act differently toward patients or patients may feel they are less intimidating and so can be asked more questions and argued with (Lorber 1985; Weisman and Teitelbaum 1985). When Candace West (1984) videotaped physician-patient encounters between 4 women and 14 men residents and women and men patients, she found that neither women nor men patients interrupted the young men physicians but did interrupt the young women physicians (p. 69). The men physicians, however, controlled the medical encounter with their interruptions when the patient was speaking.

A large-scale study of gender differences in patient-doctor interactions found that women physicians talked more than men physicians—during medical history taking, about 40 percent more—but they also gave their patients more opportunities to talk—about 58 percent more during history taking (Roter, Lipkin, and Korsgaard 1991). The researchers audiotaped 537 visits by adult patients to 101 men and 26 women physicians in a variety of primary care practice settings in 11 geographic areas in the United States and Canada. The physicians, who were in internal medicine and family practice, were predominantly young (average age was 34) and mostly white. The patients, who had made at least two previous visits to the physicians, were predominantly women (58 percent), generally poor, and older (mean age was 60), and about 45 percent were Black, Hispanic, or American Indian.

The visits with women physicians were longer than with men physicians but only by a few minutes (means of 22.9 vs. 20.3).[14] The longest visits were when women patients saw women physicians (mean, 23.3 minutes) and the shortest, when they saw men physicians (mean, 20.1). It was certain communication patterns that differed significantly. Women physicians engaged more in positive talk (described as agreements, approval, and laughter), in partnership building (asking for opinion, understanding, paraphrasing, and interpretation), in asking questions (about medical history, therapeutic regimen, emotional issues, and lifestyle), and in giving biomedical and psychosocial information.

A similar study that used videotapes of same-gender and opposite-gender interactions among 25 men and 25 women internists and 50 men and 50 women patients looked for nonverbal as well as verbal differences (Hall et al. 1994). There was little difference between the men and women physicians in social conversation, amount of technical language, emotional support, and amount of information given to patients, but the researchers found that women physicians' nonverbal communication styles were more supportive than men physicians' in that they smiled and nodded more often. In comparing patients' behavior, Hall et al. (1994) found that men and women patients spoke more to women physicians. Women patients talked an equal amount of time as the women physicians they saw because the patients offered more medical information than they did to men physicians. The women physicians encouraged their women patients' narratives with supportive statements, "uh-huhs," and nodding. In contrast, the women physicians' interactions with men patients, who were usually older than they were, presented evidence of tension and role strain:

> The [woman] physician used the least amount of technical language, smiled the most, and used voice quality that was rated as more dominant early in the visit, less friendly late in the visit, and more interested and anxious throughout. Furthermore, male patients in these interactions used voice quality that was rated as more dominant early in the visit and more bored late in the visit but also made more partnership [interactive] statements. (p. 390)

In a study by Patricia Stevens (1996), 45 lesbians, half of whom were women of color, described 332 health care encounters. Of those with men physicians, 92 percent were evaluated negatively; the same was true for only 44 percent of encounters with women physicians. Negative aspects of care were "verbal intrusion on their dignity, denigration of their intellect, and dismissal of their concerns but also . . . loss of control over bodily appearance and reproductive functioning, violation of bodily safety, and sexualization" (p. 37). A positive encounter was characterized by what was described as "solidarity: compassionate competence, empowering information exchange, and negotiated action" (p. 29). Particularly valued was "pragmatic clinical competence [combined with] sympathetic consciousness of clients' needs" (p. 29), so that medical advice was offered in a way appropriate to the client's situation. Similarly, clients wanted knowledge that would enable them to promote and maintain their own health and well-being, and they also appreciated being involved in the diagnosis and decisions about treatment.

The overall thrust of these studies of gendered doctor-patient relationships in the United States, where seeing a woman physician is a relatively new phenomenon for older patients but is expected to become more common, is that women physicians present themselves to patients as warm and supportive, which may be at odds with an image of authority and competence (Hall et al. 1994). Women patients are very relaxed with women physicians (as feminist critics of men physicians would have predicted), but men patients are not.

Because so many women physicians are in primary care, patients come to them with all their problems—major and minor illnesses, physical and emotional symptoms (Riska 1993). Physicians of either gender in office practice generally prefer similar types of patients—those who allow them to carry out their work with a minimum of fuss, who are cooperative, trusting, appreciative, and responsive to treatment (Lorber 1984:56-57). In one study, however, women physicians said they liked their patients more than men physicians did (Hall et al. 1993). The differences that patients perceive between men and women physicians may be a self-fulfilling prophecy. If patients think women physicians are more empathic, the women may in turn cultivate an expressive style to meet patients' expectations (Hall and Roter 1995). Thus, women doctors may or may not be more attuned to the "whole patient" because they are women, but if patients think they are, they may prefer a woman physician, especially for primary care. However, they may also be more dissatisfied with their care if the doctor does not live up to their gendered expectations.

When the Doctor Is a Woman

In the United States in the 19th century, women physicians specialized in the health care of women and children, set up their own clinics and hospitals, and incorporated social needs into their services.[15] The maternity clinics, for example, attended to the social difficulties of unmarried mothers. Gloria Moldow's (1987) history of Black and white women physicians in Washington, D.C., at the end of the 19th century describes medical communities segregated by race and gender. White women physicians set up their own infirmaries when they were denied access to the dispensaries and clinics that gave novice white men doctors clinical experience and contacts. The women physicians' infirmaries were run for mostly women and children patients and offered free and low-cost care. Only the Woman's Clinic, which was completely staffed by women, including a Black woman physician, survived the rise of the scientifically oriented, better equipped university hospitals, which became, in Moldow's words, "no woman's land." Through federal funding, Black men had Howard Medical School and tax-supported hospitals to work in, but few of the Black women physicians were able to attract enough patients to practice medicine full-time; many taught science in segregated high schools (Moldow, 1987).

Darlene Clark Hine's (1985) description of the lives and work of the 115 Black women who became physicians in late 19th-century America after slavery was abolished shows that many founded hospitals, nursing schools, and social service agencies as adjuncts to their private practices because none were available for the Black patients in their communities, especially in the South. They were important members of their communities—as professionals, as daughters of prominent families, and as wives of ministers, educators, and fellow doctors.

After World War I, when women got the vote in the United States they helped pass the Sheppard-Towner Act, which, in 1921, set up state and federally funded maternal and child health centers throughout the country (Barker 1993; Muncy 1991). These centers were staffed by women physicians and social workers and offered free medical services and preventive care. They also propagandized for the medicalization of childbirth and delivery by obstetricians, not midwives. By 1929, in the face of the desperate need of its members for paying patients during the Depression, the American Medical Association, dominated by men in solo, fee-for-service practice, led the fight to deny further funding to the Sheppard-Towner clinics.

In the 1960s, when Medicare and Medicaid increased the numbers of patients, the doors of U.S. medical schools and hospitals opened to women. Few women physicians determined curriculum; teaching physicians and senior residents were mostly men; and training paid little attention to the psychosocial needs or social situations of men or women patients (Harrison 1983; Scully [1980] 1994). Many of the women students followed the recommendations of their men advisers and went into obstetrics and gynecology and family practice and in time became advocates for women's health care.

In the 1970s in the United States, the feminist health movement established client-run clinics for women patients that stressed education in health matters, gynecological self-examination, and alternative medicines. Their goal was to take the control of women's bodies out of the hands of the medical system because they felt it was male dominated and oppressive (Ruzek 1978; Zimmerman 1987).[16] The problem that women patients faced, according to the feminist health movement, was twofold: a medical system that allowed patients very little control over their own care together with medical knowledge and practices that ignored many of women's needs. The cause, they argued, was a medical system dominated by men and men's values. In medical textbooks, men's bodies were the norm and women's bodies deviations from that norm (Scully and Bart 1973). Menstruation, childbirth, and menopause were considered illnesses instead of part of women's normal reproductive cycle (Martin [1987] 1992). Gynecological and obstetric practices brutalized women's bodies (Rothman 1982; Scully [1980] 1994). Physicians gave women patients too little information and rarely consulted them about their wishes before ordering hysterectomies and other drastic treatment (Fisher 1986; Todd 1989).

Although the feminist clinics preferred women to men physicians for their legally required medical backup, they were consulted as little as possible. The feminist health movement did not consider women physicians better than men physicians because they had been trained in the same pathology-oriented medical curriculum and acute-care-oriented hospitals.[17] The activists in the feminist health movement thought that by educating women patients to be more assertive and knowledgeable health consumers they would put pressure on the medical system to modify the way physicians were taught to practice:

> Implicit in the perspective of the women's health movement is the belief that if women shared control, were more centrally involved in health decision making, and brought female-oriented perspectives to balance male views, there would be changes in the environment and structure of health care that would substantially improve the health of all persons. (Zimmerman 1987:444)

The feminist health movement, the influx of women physicians into obstetrics and gynecology, and the resurgence of midwives did change pelvic examinations and birthing practices. Patients became greater participants in their prenatal care, and family-oriented birthing centers and birthing rooms in hospitals mushroomed. Drug-free deliveries and breastfeeding are encouraged to the point of being practically mandatory. However, there are still significant differences between midwives, who have a more holistic approach to pregnancy and childbirth, and obstetricians, whose focus is on pathology (Rothman 1982).[18]

By the 1990s, most of the feminist health movement's general clinics had been abandoned. The consumer movement in health care had enormously strengthened all patients' rights to question their care, but they still had to get that care through a physician-dominated system (Haug and Lavin 1983). Family practice and other primary care specialties (e.g., obstetrics and gynecology, pediatrics, and gerontology) have had an influx of resources in the United States because these general practitioners are the main workers in hospital outpatient clinics, health maintenance organizations, managed care, and other settings where doctors' fees are paid for by insurance plans or the government. As the numbers of women in medical school have increased, they have been encouraged to go into these burgeoning specialties and into primary care settings. Whether that makes for care more oriented to patients' needs is questionable (Lorber 1985). As primary care physicians in group practice or clinic settings, women physicians may seem more people oriented because first-line care is their job, but they have a fixed time to spend with patients (Riska 1993). They are not in a position to structure their delivery of health care to be sensitive to patients unless they are in their own solo or small group practices (Candib 1987, 1988).

In the past few years, women physicians in the United States have promoted research and held conferences on women's medical needs and insisted that trials of new drugs include women.[19] There is also a new doctor-oriented *Journal of Women's Health*. As director of the National Institutes of Health, Dr. Bernadine Healy set up the Office of Women's Health Research and began the Women's Health Initiative. She said that the reason she did so was not only to study the illnesses that affect women, but to look at gender differences in illnesses that affect women as well as men, such as cardiovascular disorders. These have been researched with men subjects, and only when the woman patient's symptoms emulated those of a man was she treated adequately. Healy (1991) called this problem the Yentl syndrome after the fictional 19th-century Jewish girl who disguised herself as a man in order to attend school and study the Talmud. Publications addressing women's medical needs have called physicians' attention not only to gender diversity but to the importance of within-gender variation, such as physical functioning (Nosek 1992), sexuality (Haas 1994; O'Hanlan 1995), and race and ethnicity (Allen 1994; Rosenberg, Adams-Campbell, and Palmer 1995).

The next step in attention to gender issues in health is to mainstream the knowledge about women's bodies and illness risks into general medicine, so that instead of women being seen as a deviation from the norm, the definition of what is "normal" is expanded to include women's bodies (Rosser 1994). But as is evident from the differences in the ways that women and men with heart disease are treated and the differences in the ways that women and men physicians recommend cancer-screening tests, this integrative step has not yet been taken.

Making Policy

As medicine has become a profession where authority is diluted by government regulation and income has decreased because of limitations on reimbursement, it has lost its attractiveness for men, leaving an occupational niche for women.[20] In the United States, the proportion of first-year students who are white men has declined (Jonas and Etzel 1988). Two-thirds of the Black medical students are women, as are 40 percent of the white and Asian students and 45 percent of other underrepresented racial ethnic groups (Bickel and Kopriva 1993). However, despite their increasing numbers, women physicians are unlikely to become a substantial proportion of the leadership in the near future because of a combination of institutionalized and informal sexist practices (Lorber 1993a).

The structure of work and family life still does not allow women with family responsibilities to add overtime administrative responsibilities or policy committee work to their allocated client contact hours (Lorber 1984). Women who remain single or enter into childless dual-career marriages could be formidable competitors for men with homemaker wives who allow them time to focus solely on work, but informal discriminatory practices are likely to present equally formidable barriers to their rise to the top. Women physicians without high-level administrative positions as chiefs of service in hospitals or deans of medical schools are unlikely to make any impact on the delivery of services or the production and dissemination of knowledge. The important question in assessing whether or not all types of physicians (by race, religion, social class, gender, and philosophy of practice) have equal opportunities to shape the profession depends on who has the command of resources and the authority to make policy (Freidson 1986:185-86).

Even if women physicians did run medicine as they do nursing, there is little indication that they would make it less biomedical and technological (Riska and Wegar 1993a; Todd 1989). Biochemistry and pathology of the body are the current bases of Western medical knowledge. Women and men physicians who believe that social, environmental, family, and psychological concerns should be an *integral* part of medical knowledge are not likely to restructure Western medicine until medical school curricula and training include this information.[21] Until the model of care is socio-biomedical, "medicine remains the real stuff of clinical practice unsullied by social concerns" (Fisher 1995:202).[22]

Summary

The development of Western medicine has produced a hierarchical system of caregivers, with physicians at the apex, dominating the flow of health care services to patients. As the knowledge base of medicine became rooted in the sciences (biology, biochemistry, physiology, endocrinology, and so on), the social and environmental aspects of disease and the experience of illness were given less attention in medical training and practice. The biomedical model focuses on individual pathology measured against universal norms of health and function. The supposedly normal body for a long time was that of a middle-class, young adult white man. Female physiology, including menstruation, pregnancy, and menopause, became pathology.

From a sociological perspective, the medical system is similar to the criminal justice system in that it is a way of dealing with social problems—in the case of illness, a situation in which an individual cannot fulfill normal role obligations. The individual is not blamed but is obligated to seek professional help to solve the problem and to cooperate so as to get back to the job or school or housework as soon as possible. Although many patients seek alternative caregivers, they must consult an M.D. to get prescription drugs, hospitalization, surgery, tests, and insurance reimbursement.

The structure of Western medicine is gendered because most of the physicians who are specialists, medical school educators, administrators, and policymakers are men. Women physicians are mostly in primary care. They order more tests, such as Pap smears for women patients, and have more patient-oriented communication styles. But few are in a position to change training programs and develop doctor-patient protocols for widespread use. Nurses are mostly women, and their training and practice emphasize care—attention to the patient's psychosocial as well as medical needs. However, nurses must take orders from physicians; as nurse practitioners and midwives, they are limited in the kinds of services they can offer patients.

Although most of the gender differences among health care professionals come from their positions in medical organizations, differences in communication styles, most likely an effect of life-long socialization and interaction patterns, make women physicians seem more humane than men physicians. Women physicians, like nurse practitioners, talk more to their patients about psychosocial and biomedical concerns and also offer patients more opportunities to question and argue. They thus should be preferred, since "patients clearly favor physicians who engage them personally through social conversation, who use positive language, who use partnership language, who acknowledge the patient's emotions, who discuss psychological problems, and who behave in an interested, friendly, and responsive overall manner" (Hall and Roter 1995:91). The effect, however, is to reinforce the gendered stratification of medical caregivers, with women in direct, hands-on, first-line primary care and men in prestigious and powerful specialist, administrative, and policy-making positions. It also continues the bifurcation of medical knowledge into the biological and the social (Fisher 1995). Finally, an empathic, patient-oriented practice style does not mean that the physician, woman or man, is not going to assert professional authority or that the medical encounter between physician and patient will be egalitarian (Davis 1988).

Notes

1. There is skeletal evidence from prehistoric times of successful trepanning (drilling holes in skulls to relieve pressure), bonesetting, and nutritional medications (Wood 1979).

2. According to a U.S. survey, the highest rate of use was among non-Black 25- to 49-year-olds with comparatively more education and higher income (Kessler et al. 1993).

3. Modern diagnostic technology and laboratory tests are extensions of the five senses—stethoscopes for hearing, X rays for sight, urine dipsticks for testing for sugar content (instead of tasting), sonar for touch, and so on. For the development of medical technology, see Reiser (1978).

4. For histories of the professionalization of medicine and its consequences, see Freidson 1970a, 1970b; Larson 1977; and Starr 1982.

5. In the 20th century, American medicine split along religious lines, so that large cities had Protestant, Jewish, and Catholic doctors whose patients came from the same communities. The hospitals at which these doctors practiced were supported by Protestant, Jewish, and Catholic charities (Solomon 1961).

6. Dentists have their own schools and licensing procedures. They are a parallel profession, limited to the mouth.

7. Chidambaram 1993; Elston 1993; Lorber 1993a; Notzer and Brown 1995; Riska and Wegar 1993a; Tesch et al. 1995; and Walsh 1990. The special issue of *Journal of the American Medical Women's Association*, "Gender Equity in Medicine" (September/October 1993), documents bias in specialties, salaries, practice settings, positions of authority, biomedical research, medical education, career development, and publishing.

8. For histories of nursing after Florence Nightingale, see Ashley 1976; Hine 1989; Melosh 1982; and Reverby 1987.

9. For similar findings in Scandinavia, see Kauppinen-Toropainen and Lammi 1993.

10. Feminists have criticized men's domination of science as biasing, and have also raised the same question other social constructionists of science have as to whether, as a human enterprise, scientific "facts" can ever be value free. See Birke 1986; Haraway 1988; Harding 1986, 1991; Hubbard 1990; Keller 1985; Latour 1987; Longino 1990; Restivo 1988; and Schiebinger 1989.

11. Neither Parsons nor Freidson addressed the gender implications of their analyses of the sick role; these have been teased out only later (Lorber 1975a).

12. None of the studies discussed in this section report on racial or ethnic breakdowns of physicians.

13. On breast cancer, see Kliewer and Smith 1995 and Ziegler 1993. On cervical cancer, see de Villiers et al. 1991; Reeves et al. 1989; and Seghal et al. 1993.

14. In comparing the length of encounters dealing with similar women patients seen by a man doctor and woman nurse practitioner, Fisher (1995) found considerable difference in the length of the visits—the transcript for the doctor was 8-1/2 pages long and for the nurse practitioner 40 pages (p. 50).

15. Drachman 1984; Hine 1985; Moldow 1987; Morantz and Zschoche 1980; and Morantz-Sanchez 1985.

16. The first version of *Our Bodies, Ourselves,* a Boston Women's Health Course Collective pamphlet, appeared in 1971. It was commercially published by Simon and Schuster in 1973 and has been continuously updated (see Boston

Women's Health Book Collective 1992). It was named one of the 10 most influential books in sociology of the past 25 years (Gordon and Thorne 1996). It has been translated into many languages and modified to be sensitive to women in many different cultures. Two influential pamphlets still in print that were first published in the 1970s are Ehrenreich and English 1973a, 1973b.

17. At that time, only about 11 percent of the doctors in United States were women, specializing in pediatrics, pathology, public health, and psychiatry (Lorber 1984). About a third to half the physicians in England, Europe, Scandinavia, and Israel were women, as were about 70 percent in the former Soviet Union, but they tended not to head prestigious medical institutions or make medical policy. On gender and medical education, see Martin, Arnold, and Parker 1988.

18. Pregnant women are usually allocated to obstetricians when there is a high risk of complications, but the criteria are not always objective.

19. The *Journal of the American Medical Women's Association,* official publication of the oldest association of women physicians in the United States, only recently published an issue on women and clinical trials (July/August 1994). The March/April 1995 issue discussed long-term cohort studies on women's health. For a comprehensive summary of women being included in clinical studies, see Mastroianni, Faden, and Federman 1994.

20. The number of new women students in the United States is about 40 percent, similar to England, Western Europe, and Scandinavia, but predictions are that medicine may become a woman's profession, as it has been in Russia (Riska and Wegar 1993b).

21. For the kinds of changes in medical curricula, practice, and research that could transform health-care delivery, see Dan 1994.

22. In the introductory editorial to an issue of the *Journal of the American Medical Women's Association* devoted to domestic violence and women's health, Ann Flitcraft (1996) said, "Once again we are reminded that a women's health agenda is inseparable from a women's justice agenda" (p. 76).

CHAPTER 4

If a Situation Is Defined as Real . . .

Premenstrual Syndrome and Menopause

> We should think about the consequences of defining a large proportion of
> otherwise well women as ill because of unpleasant feelings during part of
> their menstrual cycle. To assert the reality of their feelings—yes, this is
> essential—but to decide that they are abnormal and to be stamped out . . .
> that is another matter. (Laws, Hey, and Egan 1985:36)

In the 20th century, in Western culture, the menstrual cycle has been transformed
from a misunderstood and somewhat contaminating female phenomenon to a
hormonal process of puberty and preparation of the uterus for pregnancy. We
understand now that in the absence of conception, menstruation ensues; if a
sexually active woman doesn't get her monthly period, she suspects that she is
pregnant. When the eggs a woman is born with are used up, she ceases to ovulate
and secrete pregnancy-preparing hormones that thicken the lining of her uterus;
the lining no longer needs to be sloughed off in the absence of fertilization of the
ovum, and menopause occurs.[1] If there is anything a woman considers unusual
at any of the phases of the cycle, and to prevent or encourage conception, she is
urged by her family and friends to seek professional help from a doctor or another
member of the medical profession.

A medical consultation may or may not help an individual woman with her
problem, but it is likely to result in a medical label for her symptoms. From a
social perspective, the encouragement of girls and women to seek medical help
for any and all menstrual problems contaminates the status of womanhood with
the expectation of regularly recurring illness (Riessman 1983). As a result, despite
the strong evidence of women's overall physical hardiness, *all* women are considered unfit for certain kinds of work and physical activity because of their
procreative physiology. What supposedly makes females "real" women—their
menstrual cycles—makes them unreliable workers, thinkers, and leaders.

The non-Western cultural model often presents a more positive version of
menstruation, construing its phases as positive life cycle events to be ritually
celebrated (Buckley and Gottleib 1988). Chris Knight (1991) has developed a
theory that links menstruation and the origin of culture in prehistoric gathering
and hunting societies. Using Martha McClintock's (1971) observations of
menstrual synchrony among women who live together, Knight argues that since

the women of a tribe worked together, they would ovulate and menstruate at about the same time.[2] They refused to have sex with the men of the tribe during menstruation and encouraged them to go away from the camp to hunt. They induced the men to bring back the meat to be cooked with the promise of sexual relations during what would then be the women's time of greatest fertility. The symbolic taboos on menstrual blood and the blood of raw meat were, Knight argued, the origins of culture.

The more common conceptualization of menstrual taboos has been negative and oppressive of women:

> Perhaps one reason the negative image of failed production is attached to menstruation is precisely that women are in some sinister sense out of control when they menstruate. They are not reproducing, not continuing the species, not preparing to stay at home with the baby, not providing a safe, warm womb to nurture a man's sperm. (Martin [1987] 1992:47)

However, in nonindustrialized societies, menstruation does not occur as often, since women are pregnant or breastfeeding during most of their childbearing years. Menstruation is unusual, an anomaly, and it is sometimes seen as conferring magical powers; menstrual blood can be used for witchcraft—to harm or to heal (Buckley and Gottleib 1988). Close readings of ethnographic accounts reveal that it is often unclear whether menstruating women have to be kept in seclusion because they are contaminating, or others have to be kept away from menstruating women because they are sacred and frightening:

> Many menstrual taboos, rather than protecting society from a universally ascribed feminine evil, explicitly protect the perceived creative spirituality of menstruous women from the influence of others in a more neutral state, as well as protecting the latter in turn from the potent, positive spiritual force ascribed to such women. In other cultures menstrual customs, rather than subordinating women to men fearful of them, provide women with means of ensuring their own autonomy, influence, and social control. (Buckley and Gottleib 1988:7)

Whether menstruation stigmatizes or endows women with charisma, it has been seen as something that disturbs the usual social order and must be contained (Martin [1987] 1992).

In the shift to a scientific view of menstruation in the late 19th century, notions of menstrual pollution were replaced by the idea that monthly periods were necessary to women's health (Bullough and Voght 1973). In actuality, menstruating was the mark of a woman's potential fertility, and it was her childbearing capacity that had to be protected, not her health. Thus, when women began to attend college, scientific studies supposedly proved that if they used their heads too much, they would stop menstruating—they would no longer be women. There were also dire warnings that too much exercise was bad for women's fertility (Vertinsky 1990).

In the late 1970s, as women increasingly entered athletic competitions, similar scientific studies showed that women who exercised intensely would cease menstruating because they would not have enough body fat to sustain ovulation. But when one set of researchers did a year-long study that compared 66 women— 21 who were training for a marathon, 22 who ran more than an hour a week, and 23 who did less than an hour of aerobic exercise a week—they discovered that only 20 percent of the women in any of these groups had "normal" menstrual cycles every month (Prior et al. 1990).[3] The dangers of intensive training for women's fertility therefore were exaggerated as women began to compete in arenas formerly closed to them.

Emily Martin ([1987] 1992) attributes the proliferation of research on the monthly inefficiency and unreliability of women workers to the goal of keeping them out of the work force during times of high unemployment, such as during the Depression. When women workers were necessary for arms production during the World War II, other studies (sometimes by the same researchers) showed that menstruation was no hindrance to women doing any kind of work.

According to many feminists, the subordinate social status of women is the result of historic and economic processes; biology is used as a pervasive justification for their subordination but is not the cause of it (Delaney, Lupton, and Toth 1977; Koeske 1983; Lorber 1993b).[4] Gloria Steinem asked in 1978, "What would happen . . . if suddenly, magically, men could menstruate and women could not? . . . The answer is clear—menstruation would become an enviable, boast-worthy, masculine event" (p. 110).

In 1993, in a long article in *The Quarterly Review of Biology*, Margie Profet, a woman evolutionary biologist, presented a new biological theory of why women menstruate. Profet argued that "the function of menstruation is to defend against pathogens transported to the uterus by sperm" (p. 338). Using data from research on the menstrual cycles of primates and other animals where fertilization is internal, she claimed that the design of the uterus and the nonclotting quality of menstrual blood are evidence of menstruation's protective function in ridding the uterus of potentially harmful bacteria. Her theory countered the underlying assumptions of the old folk view—that women are impure and menstruation gets rid of their impurities. In symbolic terms, her new theory transfers the notion of impurity to men.

The social construction of the menstrual cycle has not disappeared with greater knowledge of the physiology of the female reproductive system. At present, in medical and popular publications, the divisions of the cycle differ in number, transition points, markers, and names:

> Not only are there discrepancies over how many phases constitute "the menstrual cycle" and what to call these supposedly distinct phases, but there is also contention in the literatures over how long some of these stages should last, particularly "ovulation," "postovulation," "premenstruation," "menstruation," and perhaps most importantly, the whole "menstrual cycle." (Foster 1996:535)

The 28-day cycle, which Johanna Foster (1996) says is a widely accepted myth in our culture, is based on an equally conventional month of four 7-day weeks, not on a lunar month, which takes 29.5 days (pp. 536-37). The "facts" are always social facts, specific to a time, place, and culture; values and meaning are sometimes explicit, sometimes assumed.[5] The controversy over PMS (premenstrual syndrome), for example, has focused on a part of the cycle that was previously ignored. The biomedical perspective on the physical, behavioral, and emotional effects of the menstrual cycle is thus a social construction, built out of the values of our time.

Medicalizing Menstruation

Because Western medicine defines menstruation as a normal physiological process, part of the cycle of female puberty and procreation, girls are not expected to consult a doctor or nurse when they get their first periods unless the menses are unusually early or late or accompanied by severe cramps or other problems. However, the definitions of "early," "late," "severe," "cramps," and "problems" take on a medical coloration because the body and its functioning is the domain of medicine in Western cultures (Bransen 1992; Scambler and Scambler 1993). Articles on menstrual problems in women's magazines are written by doctors or cite doctors, and the accounts of women's experiences in them reflect the biomedical view that these problems are individualized abnormalities caused by imbalanced hormones (Chrisler and Levy 1990; Markens 1996).

In the 20th century, two syndromes (sets of symptoms) have emerged into popular and medical discourse: premenstrual syndrome (or PMS) and the menopause. PMS is linked to the monthly cycle of menstruation and the menopausal syndrome to the gradual cessation of regular menstrual cycles. The onset, occurrence, and cessation of menstruation are caused by hormonal shifts that are, in themselves, normal physiological events but that can have diverse bodily and behavioral effects. The question is, why are these accompanying effects considered "symptoms"? And is the translation of diffuse "feelings" into a clear "diagnosis" benign or detrimental? The answer to the first question depends on a woman's culture and the extent to which the menstrual cycle is medicalized in her social world. The answer to the second question depends on how diagnoses of PMS and menopause are viewed in medical as well as lay discourse.

The current view of PMS and menopause as producing uncontrollable emotions and behavior is reminiscent of the view of pollution as that which disturbs the social order (Douglas 1966). As Sophie Laws says,

> The "symptoms" of [PMS] which the doctors show most concern over—depression, anxiety, and so on—are mental states which do not "fit" with women's culturally created notions of ourselves as nice, kind, gentle, etc. "Mood change," as such, is often listed as a symptom—demonstrating that change *as such* is not culturally acceptable. . . . There's just no room for women

to have strong feelings of their own, disrupting this comfortable flow of emotional services. (Laws et al. 1985:35)

In this sense, PMS and the menopause have replaced menstruation itself as an antisocial force that needs to be subdued. To counter this view, some feminists have reinterpreted menstrually related mood swings as having positive rather than negative effects, describing, for example, premenstrual tension as a heightened energy state (Guinan 1988).

Although there certainly are women who could benefit from amelioration of disabling menstrual conditions, they are not necessarily the majority (Yankauskas 1990). Nonetheless, all women are said to suffer (and make others suffer in turn) from the "horrors" of "that time of month" or "that time of life." In our society, these syndromes denigrate women as a group and justify their subordinate social status (Laws 1983; Rittenhouse 1991; Zita 1988). In this chapter, I intend to show how PMS and the menopause came to be medical syndromes and what the social consequences have been. To paraphrase a classic statement of sociology, "If a situation is defined as real, it is real in its consequences."[6]

Premenstrual Syndrome: "Hormonal Hurricane" or High-Energy State?[7]

Premenstrual tension was described and attributed to hormonal causes over 65 years ago (Frank 1931); since then, most research has followed the biomedical model—defining it as *a* syndrome, with *a* hormonal cause, *a* pathology located in the *individual.* Much of the medical and lay focus has been on the psychological aspects of what was called Late Luteal Phase Dysphoric Disorder and Premenstrual Dysphoric Disorder in the American Psychiatric Association's official diagnostic manuals (Figert 1995; Gitlin and Pasnau 1989). These psychological effects are seen as problems when they interfere with a woman's capacity to carry on her normal social functions, when they disturb her social relationships, and most notoriously, when they cause violent acting out (Rittenhouse 1991). Critics have noted that there is considerable confusion about what is more familiarly called PMS—whether it is a single syndrome, when it occurs, whether hormones cause the psychological effects, how many women have debilitating effects, and whether the effects are necessarily negative.[8]

The diffuseness and multiplicity of symptoms are indications of diagnostic slipperiness—close to 100 different symptoms of PMS have been listed (Laws et al. 1985:37-38). Some women experience premenstrual bodily changes, others emotional ups and downs, and still others a combination of both, all in mild, moderate, and severe forms:

> The emotional states most commonly reported in studies of PMS are tension, anxiety, depression, irritability, and hostility. Somatic complaints include abdominal bloating, swelling, breast tenderness, headache, and backache. Behavioral changes frequently reported are an avoidance of social contact, a

change in work habits, increased tendency to pick fights (especially with a spouse/partner or children), and crying spells. (Abplanalp 1983:109)

Many women have mild symptoms (just as many women have mild menstrual discomfort); the incidence of severe syndromes (or debilitating menstrual periods) is much less common (Golub 1992).

There is some question about the cyclicity of PMS. Many women and men experience mood swings based on the day of the week; for women, these may modify or intensify menstrual-cycle mood swings (Hoffmann 1982; Rossi and Rossi 1977). Mary Brown Parlee (1982b) found that individual women were less likely to attribute psychological mood swings to menstrual cycles than to other causes, such as reactions to difficulties at work or at home; when the data were grouped, however, the presence of menstrual mood cycles was magnified because the other patterns were idiosyncratic. Daily self-reports gave "a picture of what might be called a 'premenstrual elation syndrome' that is the opposite of the negative one embodied in the stereotype of premenstrual tension" (Parlee 1982b:130). Retrospective reports from these same women described their feelings in stereotypical terms.

Stereotypically, women suffering from PMS are said to be cranky, irritable, angry, violent, and out of control. These characteristics assume some kind of comparison—with the same woman at other times of the month or with the way women are supposed to be. One woman physician sardonically commented that perhaps the effects of what is defined as premenstrual syndrome—anger and irritability—stand out because this behavior is in contrast to three weeks of pleasant sociability (Guinan 1988). Sharon Golub (1992) suggests that comparisons with men would be useful:

> While women's moods may vary cyclically, there is no evidence that women are more prone to anger than men. In fact, the opposite is probably true. Witness the far higher rates of crime and accidents among men. Some have suggested that the worst part of being premenstrual is that that is when women are most like men. (p. 204)

Control groups, however, are rarely used in research on PMS (Fausto-Sterling 1985:106-7). Samples are usually not diversified on race, religion, social class, or age, nor are cycles followed for a long period of time. Subjective feelings of tension, agitation, depression, and anger are loosely defined and poorly measured. The menstrual cycle is assumed to be the cause of mood changes, never the other way around, even though research has shown that hormones are as affected by behavior as behavior is by hormones (Kemper 1990; Koeske 1983). The notorious connection between premenstrual tension and crimes, suicides, and other destructive actions may be due to emotional stress that causes changes both in the menstrual cycle and pathological behavior. Parlee (1982a) found that women taking important examinations are as likely to be premenstrual or menstruating as women committing crimes are.

The controversy over whether PMS could be used as a defense in murder trials made the syndrome a household word in 1981 (Laws 1983). An equally contentious battle went on during the late 1980s over whether to make PMS an official diagnosis in the revised third edition of the *Diagnostic and Statistical Manual of Mental Disorders* (*DSM-III-R*), which delayed its publication by two years (Figert 1995). In this battle, the feminist Committee on Women of the American Psychiatric Association enlisted professional and lay women's groups to prevent the legitimation of a diagnosis that they felt had the potential of stigmatizing all menstruating women as potentially "crazy." They argued that even a careful definition that emphasized severity and intractability of psychological reactions to a primarily physiological phenomenon was likely to be misconstrued as constantly recurring instability and irrationality. However, without an official diagnosis, third-party insurers would not pay for treatment of PMS as a primary psychiatric disorder.

The issue of who was to treat PMS was interwoven with the question of the definition of the disorder (Figert 1995). If the problem is due to hormonal imbalance, then it is the province of gynecologists; if the problem is primarily emotional, then it should be treated by psychiatrists. Psychologists, social workers, and other mental health workers who were not M.D.s claimed the right to treat what they defined as a social situational problem. Feminist women's groups pushed for self-treatment and alternative health-care remedies of the discomforts of a normal physiological process. The Institute for Research on Women's Health in Washington, D.C., using feminist networks and the mailing list of the National Coalition for Women's Mental Health, focused media and the public's attention on the issue and encouraged a letter-writing campaign to the APA.

The outcome was a compromise—a listing in the Appendix of the *DSM-III-R* and also in the *DSM-IV*, the manual's latest edition. Such placement indicates that the syndrome needs additional research for verification and use as an insurable diagnosis. It was a defeat for the professional and lay women who wanted to keep PMS out of the manual entirely, Figert (1995) argues, and a victory for the PMS researchers who wanted criteria to make their research "more definable, specific, and fundable" (p. 68). But the criteria (physical and psychological, not social situational) then shape the way the research is designed and predicts the ultimate outcome (medical or psychological treatment, not changes in relationships or lifestyle). As Parlee (1994) points out, the call for more rigorous criteria of menstrual cycles frequently means that even in social scientists' research, physiological measurements of hormonal levels are built into the research design, necessitating collaboration with biomedically trained researchers (p. 98).

Although positive mood changes have been reported for over a decade, they are almost never looked for in most PMS research (Martin [1987] 1992:128-29; Parlee 1982b). Martin ([1987] 1992) suggests that from a feminist perspective, premenstrual tension can be positive—not only a release of ordinarily suppressed anger at the everyday put-downs women are subject to, but a different kind of consciousness, concentration, and creativity: "Does the loss of ability to concentrate mean a greater ability to free-associate? Loss of muscle control, a gain in ability to relax? Decreased efficiency, increased attention to a smaller number of tasks?" (p. 128). Women who have autonomy in their work could find these times productive, but factory workers, data processors, nurses, and mothers of small children—the majority of women—cannot afford the loss of self-discipline. Given the way that work and time are organized in industrialized societies, "women are perceived as malfunctioning and their hormones out of balance rather than the organization of society and work perceived as in need of a transformation to demand less constant discipline and productivity" (Martin [1987] 1992:123). Since work and family life are not likely to be reorganized, women who are overwhelmed by the pressures of their daily lives may find it necessary to claim illness periodically as a means of getting relief without blame (Parlee 1994:104-5).

Menopause: The End of Womanhood
or the Beginning of a Valued Status?

As with PMS, the biomedical aspects of menopause have outweighed its social factors in professional and lay discourse (Bell 1990). Western culture imposes a negative connotation on women's experiences of their bodies and a separation of body and mind. Western women are given no chance to contemplate their bodies as located in time and place and as *theirs* to control (Levesque-Lopman 1988). Menopause has become a sign of woman's aging, the end of her procreative capabilities. Since women's social status in our society is so intertwined with her body and biology, menopause has been seen as virtually the end of womanhood (Zita 1993). In contrast, Peruvian women gain full adulthood around the time of menopause, reaping social and financial benefits and freedom from daily chores and from large extended families (Barnett 1988).

Affluent men or those who have attained secure positions in academe or other professions had, in the past, not worried as much about aging as middle-class women, but their cultural protections may be disappearing. The depressed economy and women's growing financial and psychological independence make men vulnerable to the marketing of facelifts and other cosmetic surgery, hair transplants and dyes, and exercise and sports regimens (Gullette 1993). Despite talk of a male climacteric, the markers of aging in men are not medicalized, as menopause is. So the pressures on men to "do something about aging" are less likely to be backed by a powerful medical ideology that translates natural processes into illness and routinizes hormonal replacement therapy in the name of "feminine forever."[9] No one seems to be arguing that men over 50 are not masculine.

What makes menopause different from PMS is that the condition itself, not just its effects, is seen as a medical problem. Cessation of menstruation, the result of no longer ovulating, has become a "deficiency disease" to be cured by permanent hormone replacement therapy (McCrea 1986). The use of estrogen, popularized in the 1960s, was supposed to cure psychological as well as physiological effects of menopause—to energize, tranquilize, counteract depression, increase libido, alleviate hot flashes, minimize night sweating, and reverse vaginal dryness. By the mid-1970s, the danger of endometrial cancer led to medical recommendations that estrogen be used only for symptoms directly related to lower hormone levels (body temperature fluctuations and vaginal changes), at low doses, and for a short period of time. Instead, drug companies came up with an estrogen-progesterone combination that they claimed was safer, although there have still been reports of incidences of breast cancer with its use (Lewis 1993). Around the same time, a new reason for extended use emerged— preventing the loss of bone mass and forestalling the possible development of osteoporosis (Klinge 1996). An additional indication for long-term hormone replacement that is currently being debated is prevention of heart disease (Jonas and Manolio 1996; Nachtigall and Nachtigall 1995).

Early studies of symptoms of menopause were done on women who had sought medical help or who had had hysterectomies. To track the occurrence of perimenopausal, menopausal, and postmenopausal symptoms in a more general population, a cohort of 2,572 women, aged 45-55 in 1981, were selected from census lists in 38 Massachusetts cities and towns (Avis and McKinlay 1991, 1995).[10] The sample was diversified by size of city or town, per capita income, and race. The women were interviewed for 30 minutes by telephone every nine months over five years. At each interview, they were asked questions about their menstrual status, physical health, utilization of health care, and sociodemographic status. On a rotating basis, they were asked about their social support networks, their lifestyle (including depression), and their help-seeking behavior.

This carefully constructed survey found that "natural menopause seems to have no major impact on health or health behavior. The majority of women do not seek additional help concerning menopause, and their attitudes toward it are, overwhelmingly, positive or neutral" (Avis and McKinlay 1995:45). Almost 69 percent of the women reported not being bothered by hot flashes or night sweats, and 23 percent reported not having had them at all. Only 32 percent said they had consulted a doctor for menopausal-related symptoms, and these women were likely to have been depressed before menopause. The authors conclude that the stressful impact of other life events far outweighs the stress of menopause.

Other studies have also shown that the incidence of supposedly universal symptoms of menopause are not experienced by every woman. Japanese women are much less likely to report experiencing hot flashes or night sweats during the year following cessation of their menses than Canadian women in Manitoba and U.S. women in Massachusetts (Lock 1993:36).[11] Interviews with 603 postmenopausal Indonesian women found that less than a third reported having had hot flashes; they used an herbal drink and daily servings of papaya (which is estrogenic) as a remedy for hot flashes and for vaginal dryness (Flint and Samil 1990). A Netherlands study of 4,426 women and 4,253 men between the ages of 25 and 75 used data from a general health questionnaire administered to a sample of general practitioners' patients (Van Hall, Verdel, and Van Der Velden 1994). The researchers found that the only symptom directly related to menopause was excessive perspiration. Diffuse complaints, such as dizziness, headache, tiredness, nervousness, sleeplessness, listlessness, palpitations, aggressiveness, irritability, and depression were neither gender specific nor age specific. Van Hall et al. (1994) concluded that "there is no rationale in prescribing estrogens for psychologic problems or mood disorders occurring during the climacteric or the postmenopausal period" (p. 47).

Margaret Lock's (1993) study of menopause in Japan found that it was not medicalized:

> The dominant physicians' discourse, which they share with nearly all their patients, remains one in which *konenki* figures as a natural transition, one through which both men and women must pass, but during which, because of their biological makeup, women are thought to be more vulnerable than men to physical and emotional difficulties. (p. 293)

A visit to a physician is encouraged for women only to check that there are no other health problems, and hormonal replacement therapy is used very conservatively; herbal medicine is preferred. Without widespread use of hormonal replacement, Japanese women have one-quarter the mortality rate from heart disease and half the incidence of osteoporosis of North American Caucasian women, despite a less dense bone mass; their life expectancy is the longest in the world (pp. 295-96).

If menstrual cycles supposedly cause so much difficulty for women, why, asks Sharon Golub (1992), isn't the cessation of menstruation more welcome? Her answer is "fear: fear of aging, fear of loss of sexuality, fear of getting depressed, fear of loss of health" (p. 236). Yet when these connotations of menopause are teased apart, the health aspect elicits more negative attitudes than when menopause is construed as a sign of aging, like gray hair and retirement, or when it is seen as a life transition, like puberty and leaving home (Gannon and Ekstrom 1993). Furthermore, women on the other side of the menstrual divide, those who are a year past their last period, have expressed very positive feelings—"of beginning a new life, of feeling great, of being wonderful, and of enjoying their lives" (Dickson 1990:27). The study of postmenopausal Indonesian women also found a high incidence of reports of positive feelings—affection, excitement, well-being, energy, and orderliness (Flint and Samil 1990).

Feminist analyses look beyond the individual to sociocultural phenomena—the social status of older women, differing images of sexuality for women and men, and place in a constellation of family and friends.[12] These phenomena, which vary from culture to culture and by race and class in the United States, structure the experience of menopause. Thus, aging women in the United States are supposed to turn to their doctors for help; in Japan, they expect to be looked after by their daughters-in-law (Lock 1993:386). Among upper-caste women in India who are segregated from men, menopause lifts their restrictions and gives them the freedom to socialize outside the home and to travel (Flint 1982). For American women, "it meant pleasure at avoiding whatever discomfort they felt during periods and relief from the nuisance of dealing with bleeding, pads, or tampons. . . . For those women sexually active with men, it meant delight to not suffer the fear of pregnancy" (Martin [1987] 1992:175)—but not an elevation to a more valued status.

Jacquelyn Zita's (1993) suggestion for Western women is to "bring all aged crones into view, not as spectral shadows, but as women in our full presence, substance, and power" (p. 75). Germaine Greer's (1991) manifesto is even more confrontational: "Though the old woman is both feared and reviled, she need not take the intolerance of others to heart, for women over fifty already form one of the largest groups in the population structure of the Western world" (p. 4).

Politics of PMS and Menopause

Reviewing her own 20 years of work on menstruation, the conferences she has attended, and the proliferating literature on PMS, Mary Brown Parlee (1994) concludes that

> biomedical researchers' knowledge claims . . . have come to prevail over those of social scientists. . . . As in the popular culture, biomedical literature now routinely and unproblematically (incontestably) refers to PMS as some*thing* some women "have." Permitted scientific disputes now concern what causes "it" and how "it" can be treated. (p. 103)

The same thing, she suggests, has happened to menopause. In both instances, drug companies profit from enormous markets for their products; gynecologists profit from expansion of their practices in a time of declining births; psychiatrists (especially those in managed care) also benefit from a larger pool of patients; and physician researchers' quantifiable projects get funds from government agencies, medical centers, and drug companies.

The biomedical model of PMS and menopause even has advantages for women. In the late 19th century, middle- and upper-class women could use the sick role as a way of opting out of the obligation to bear numerous children and run households to suit their husband's wishes; in the late 20th century, women can get time out and attention to their needs with a diagnosis of menstrual complications legitimated by the ultimate authority, the physician (Ehrenreich and English 1973b; Parlee 1994). For working-class women with access to medical care, who had no such recourse in the 19th century, medical attention may be better than no attention.

What is wrong with a medical diagnosis of PMS and menopause?[13] First, it results in treatment with hormones, drugs, and tranquilizers, which can have debilitating and dangerous side effects. Second, it objectifies and pathologizes women's bodies and the menstrual cycle. Third, it focuses attention only on the negative aspects, the concomitant discomforts and emotional upsets that bring a woman to the doctor, and ignores the positive aspects frequently reported in field surveys. Fourth, it makes women "double deviants"— they are ill periodically and cannot be blamed for their symptoms, but their reputations as reliable workers, and especially their potential for positions of authority, are seriously damaged. And finally, women's anger and protest over the conditions of their lives are safely defused by a diagnosis that can be contained within the medical system.

Transforming Diagnoses Back Into Women's Troubles

Because so much of the current perspective on PMS and menopause is biomedical, it is important to look at what goes on in the doctor's office that turns presenting symptoms into medical diagnoses. In her analysis of medical encounters between women patients and men doctors, Kathy Davis (1988) describes how patients' emotionally loaded reports of diffuse complaints are shaped and focused into treatable medical syndromes by doctors who are genuinely trying to ameliorate the patient's distress. Her accounts suggest the process by which women's search for help for disturbances of the body and emotions around the times of menstruation and its cessation get turned into PMS and the menopause.

In presenting their reasons for coming to the doctor, Davis notes, patients not only describe their symptoms or the progress of an ongoing illness but also complain about their troubles, their suffering, and their distress:

> Patients defined their problems as part of the activity of complaining rather than as a complaint, as an experience rather than a diagnostic category, as something serious enough to feel bad about, and themselves as persons deserving both sympathy and respect. (p. 333)

The physician's task is to use medical expertise to sort out what is significant in the patient's "story about trouble." The physician could tell the patient that she had no treatable medical condition and just listen for the time allotted for the visit. But physicians are trained to "do something," and so they adapt patients' presenting complaints to fit the most likely medical diagnosis and urge the patients to accept it and the treatment that goes with it.

The encounter, Davis (1988) notes, is not one of overt power and coercion. The patient comes to the doctor as an expert for help with something she feels she cannot handle on her own. The doctor, in turn, feels obligated to offer practical help. Since the physician's perspective and knowledge are biomedical, the patient's troubles are transformed into a medical diagnosis. What is medically significant is the patient's physiological or psychosomatic reactions and not her social situation or social status. The remedy is a prescription for medication, not help in understanding what is wrong in the patient's life or support for doing something about her troubles herself. "Not only were the women's problems shorn of their contextuality and forced into professional schemes of relevance, but the GP seemed unable, in many cases, to understand what made the problems problematic in the first place" (p. 345).

Although Davis did not have a comparison group of women physicians, Sue Fisher's (1995) work on the similarities and differences of women patients' medical encounters with men physicians and women nurse practitioners suggests that even health care workers committed to a caring style maintain asymmetrical power, set the limits of appropriate topics for discussion, and pressure for compliance with what they think is the best treatment. The nurse practitioners do, however, pay much more attention to patients' accounts of their lifestyles and current social situations, grant more competence and knowledge to their patients as women, and are less likely to reproduce conventional ideas about appropriate feminine roles and behavior. They also tend to suggest treatments tailored to patients' specific needs.

Women physicians are located between men physicians and women nurse practitioners in the medical hierarchy. Unless they have set up a consciously feminist and patient-oriented practice, they may act no differently than men toward women patients (Lorber 1985). However, as was found in the research discussed in Chapter 3, women physicians do listen and talk more. They are, however, likely to use medical diagnoses of menopausal problems and suggest treatment by drugs or hormones (Bush 1992). However, even within the medical system, a different perspective means different medical practices. Thus, if uterine bleeding removes pathogens, Profet (1993) recommends that it should not be suppressed when it is nonmenstrual; treatment should focus only on the source of the infection. She also recommends that diaphragms or condoms be used by sexually active women who are pregnant, menopausal, or amenorrheic for reasons other than having had a hysterectomy.[14]

It is probable that only by going outside the conventional medical system can menstrual discomforts be demedicalized. Alternative healing practices, such as diet, massage, exercise, and nutritional and herbal remedies, may be more appropriate to the diffuse and periodic symptoms so embedded in a woman's daily life than the hormones and tranquilizers doctors are likely to prescribe (Harrison 1985).[15] But the search for treatment does not resolve the larger question of why the subtle or marked physical and emotional changes that accompany menstrual cycles are considered abnormal and social problems and not part of normal variations in the rhythm of days, weeks, months, and years. For that, a different perspective is needed, one that is fully aware of gender issues, as well as the accompanying effects of race, ethnicity, social class, marital status, parental responsibilities, work pressures, and all the other situational aspects of women's lives:

> If we are to respect ourselves as women we have to own all our states of being
> as parts of ourselves, even, and perhaps especially, the painful ones. If we are
> angry or sad before our periods, there is anger or sadness in us, and there are
> reasons for it. The menstrual cycle does not impose extraneous problems on
> a woman—it is part of her. (Laws et al. 1985:57-58)

Summary

In this chapter, I have argued that a biomedical focus on menstruation, currently the perspective legitimated by medicine and scientific research, can have negative consequences for individual women and for the status of women in Western society. Medical attention turns diffuse physiological and psychological symptoms that occur premenstrually and around the time of cessation of menses into discrete syndromes—PMS and the menopause. Reports in the scientific and lay media ignore positive feelings—elation, energy, and well-being—frequently reported in surveys and interviews of women who do not consult doctors.

The social construction of PMS and menopause as medical syndromes and not as part of normal physiological functions has made PMS into psychological pathology and menopause into a deficiency disease. Construing PMS as a condition of irritability at best and irrationality at worst puts an individual woman into a stigmatized sick role for a week every month. The social status of women in general is contaminated because PMS is used as a validation of their purported unreliability as skilled workers and especially their supposed ineffectiveness in positions of authority.

Construing menopause as a deficiency disease has led, in the United States, to widespread prescriptions of long-term hormonal replacement therapy for specific symptoms, such as hot flashes, night sweats, and vaginal dryness; for diffuse symptoms, such as depression, sleeplessness, fatigue, and sexual disinterest; and for prevention of heart disease and osteoporosis. For an individual woman, short-term hormonal use might be a useful remedy for extremely discomforting symptoms, but long-term use carries the risk of breast and uterine cancer. For women in general, the connotation of menopause as a lack of the crucial mark of womanhood (potential for procreation) undercuts the status of older women as full human beings.

Cross-cultural and cross-national studies give evidence of contrasting views of menstruating women and women who have completed their childbearing. In some cultures, menstruating women have an aura of spiritual and creative power. Similarly, in countries that mark the passage of life transitions ritually and socially, menarche and menstruation are important events in that they change a woman's status—from child to marriageable woman and from mother to respected elder.

Feminist critiques of the biomedical model of menstruation have focused on its negative use in rationalizing the subordinate status of women in Western society. They have also publicized the potential risks and side effects of long-term therapy with tranquilizers and hormones as well as the stigmatizing consequences of labeling all women as periodically incapacitated or insane. Without denigrating the discomforts and debilities some women experience, they have recommended short-term specific use of medical remedies and the effectiveness of alternative medicine. They have also argued that research on the social-psychological and situational aspects of menstruation would produce fuller knowledge of women's feelings and behavior at "that time of month" and "that time of life."

Notes

1. Not all cycles are ovulatory; anovulatory cycles are common when menses first start and as they are stopping (Foster 1996).

2. For other studies on menstrual synchrony, see Golub 1992.

3. According to Scambler and Scambler (1993), a 28-day cycle is barely the mode and not necessarily "normal."

4. Parlee (1994) feels that it is not a coincidence that widespread attention began to be paid to PMS as a prevalent woman's illness at the same time that feminism became a significant social movement (p. 101).

5. Donna Haraway (1981) said, "Facts are theory laden; theories are value laden; values are history laden" (p. 477).

6. The exact phrasing of the sociological theorem, from a book by W. I. Thomas and Dorothy Swaine Thomas (1927), is "If men define situations as real, they are real in their consequences" (p. 47).

7. Fausto-Sterling (1985) used the phrase "hormonal hurricanes" in her chapter on menstruation, the menopause, and female behavior.

8. Abplanalp 1983; Fausto-Sterling 1985; Figert 1995; Koeske 1983; Laws 1983, 1990; Laws, Hey, and Egan 1985; Lennane and Lennane 1973; Martin [1987] 1992; Parlee 1973, 1982a, 1994; Rittenhouse 1991; and Zita 1988.

9. *Feminine Forever* was the name of the book popularizing estrogen use written by Robert Wilson (1966), a gynecologist from New York City who had set up a foundation to promote estrogen that was supported by over $1 million in grants from the pharmaceutical industry (McCrea 1986: 297). The popular literature at the time estrogen was first widely used in menopause was blunt in its description of the postmenopausal woman. The author of *Everything You Wanted to Know about Sex but Were Afraid to Ask* said in the 1969 edition, "Not really a man but no longer a functional woman, these individuals live in the world of intersex" (quoted in Fausto-Sterling 1985:111).

10. The standard epidemiological definition of natural menopause is 12 consecutive months of amenorrhea with no other cause; perimenopause is defined as a change in cycle regularity or periods of amenorrhea of 11 months or less (Avis and McKinlay 1995:46).

11. Comparative statistics on percentage rates of hot flashes and night sweats, respectively, are the following:

    Japan—15.2 and 3 of 1,104

    Manitoba—41.5 and 22.2 of 1,039

    Massachusetts—43.9 and 11.3 of 5,505

12. Callahan 1993; Greer 1991; Lock 1993; Martin [1987] 1992; and Voda, Dinnerstein, and O'Donnell 1982.

13. These criticisms can be found in the writers in notes 8 and 12.

14. Only condoms prevent infection from bacterial and viral infections.

15. One of the most famous remedies for "female complaints" was Lydia E. Pinkham's Vegetable Compound. First marketed in 1875 out of Mrs. Pinkham's home in Massachusetts, it was manufactured for 100 years (Stage 1979).

CHAPTER 5

A Modern Plague

Gender and AIDS

> And the gay disease, which came to be known as ... AIDS slowly ate its
> way through those new populations, women and their children, hidden
> and quiet and savage. (Nechas and Foley 1994:88)

When AIDS (acquired immunodeficiency disease) surfaced in the United States
in 1981, it was an epidemic in the population of urban, gay, mostly white middle-
and upper-class men. Thought to be caused by promiscuity and high living, it
was called GRID (gay-related immune disease). Today, throughout the world,
AIDS is an epidemic of poor, urban men and women, most of whom are Black,
Hispanic, or Asian, and primarily heterosexual in their relationships. It is known
to be caused by a virus, HIV-1, which enters the cells of the immune system and
destroys their capability to fight diseases. Although people may live for years
with the HIV virus in their bodies, those whose immune systems are severely
weakened get incurable disorders, such as pneumonia, blindness, diarrhea, and
brain deterioration (the symptoms of full-blown AIDS), from which they die.
Combinations of drugs have delayed the development of AIDS symptoms and
produced remissions, but the regimen is complicated and expensive.

Tracking by the U.S. Centers for Disease Control (CDC) began in 1981, but it
took years before the persistent medical reports of a strange pneumonia and a
rare cancer among young, gay men received any response from governments
(Shilts 1987). One case of a woman with a similar syndrome was reported to the
CDC in 1981, and there was a medical report in 1982 on opportunistic infections
in four women drug users and in a bisexual woman with a male drug-using
partner (Masur et al. 1982; Nechas and Foley 1994:87). In 1982 and 1983, Joyce
Wallace and her colleagues reported similar blood-level markers of HIV infection
in men who had sex with men and in women sex workers in New York City, but
despite a continuous stream of such reports, it took longer than it did for gay men
before the medical profession acknowledged that women were vulnerable to
AIDS and needed help (Corea 1992; Nechas and Foley 1994; Patton 1994; Wallace
et al. 1982, 1983). There were numerous medical reports that the symptoms of
women with AIDS were different from those of men, but it took protests at AIDS
conferences and a lawsuit against the U.S. Social Security Administration before
the CDC changed the list of diagnostic signs of AIDS, adding recurrent and

virtually untreatable vaginal yeast infection and invasive cervical cancer.[1] Before that change, women who were dying of AIDS-related opportunistic infections that didn't fit the male pattern were denied AIDS-targeted disability and medical benefits (Corea 1992).[2]

The focus of attention in clinical trials and the mass media has been on women's potential to infect men and babies, not on their potential to be infected (Corea 1992; Patton 1994). Yet in heterosexual relationships, women are more vulnerable than men—the male-to-female rate of transmission is much higher than the female-to-male rate (Campbell 1995; Chu et al. 1992; Padian et al. 1987, 1991). In heterosexual couples where only one partner is HIV positive, it is more often the man than the woman. Three-quarters of the women who are HIV positive at the time of delivery do *not* pass the virus to their children: The maternal-infant transmission rate is about 25-30 percent; with drug treatment during pregnancy, it can be reduced to about 8 percent (Connor et al. 1994).

Risk of exposure is embedded in the gender politics of heterosexual, bisexual, and homosexual relationships: The more intimate the relationship, the less frequently condoms are used. Sexually active adolescents, both boys and girls, are now showing elevated rates of HIV infection amid arguments over condom distribution and masturbation (DiClemente 1990). In Africa, India, and Asia, the paths of transmission follow truck drivers, sex workers, and women and men migrants to urban areas. In Western countries, the practice of friends and lovers sharing needles has linked HIV infection and AIDS closely to intravenous drug use. The controversy over mandatory testing of pregnant women and newborns is ongoing, and there have been fears of forced abortions and sterilization of those women who are HIV positive (Beckerman et al., 1996).

In this chapter, I focus on the current social context of HIV transmission and the health care of those with AIDS. Using a gender analysis, I discuss the risks of getting and transmitting HIV, the care and social support for those who are HIV positive and those who have symptoms of AIDS, and the implications of the social and cultural construction of the infection and the disease.[3]

AIDS by the Numbers

According to the statistics reported to the United Nations in June 1996 and to the 11th International Conference on AIDS in July 1996, about 42 percent of the estimated 21 to 22 million adults throughout the world who are HIV positive are women, and their numbers are increasing rapidly in every region (Altman 1996a, 1996b). In sub-Saharan African countries, where 14 million HIV-positive people account for 64 percent of the worldwide total, more women than men are infected. The spread of HIV infection in Africa, Asia, India, the Caribbean, and Latin America has been by heterosexual intercourse (Altman 1996b; Shenon 1996). Marriage and long-term relationships are no protection, for partners may be drug users who share needles or who may have sexual relationships with other men or other women (Navarro 1995). Another source of heterosexual transmission is from a partner who has been infected through a blood transfusion. Almost all the hemophiliacs who were infused with blood-clotting factors between the mid-1970s and the mid-1980s are HIV positive (Kolata 1991). Most of these are married men, and a high percentage of their wives are also infected (Patton 1994).

In the United States, according to data from the CDC, AIDS was the leading cause of death among men, ages 25 to 44, in 1992 (Altman 1995b). Among women in this age group, it was fourth, behind cancer, unintentional injuries, and heart disease, but 1995 estimates were that AIDS is expected to be the second leading cause of death for women in the United States in a year or two. It is seventh for children.

These AIDS statistics are counts of those reported to be HIV positive or who are treated for diseases to which their compromised immune systems make them vulnerable.[4] What the statistics do not tell us is just how widespread HIV infection actually is (Altman 1994). The latency period from infection with the virus to the development of symptoms of AIDS is said to be an average of 11.5 years, but there are people who tested positive for HIV but did not develop symptoms for 15 or 20 years (Altman 1995a). Cases of AIDS are turning up among people over 60 (Paauw, Spach, and Wallace 1993). There is a debate over the extent of HIV infection and AIDS among lesbians (Goldstein 1995; Gómez 1995). Thus, besides cases not reported as AIDS related, there are HIV-positive people who have never been tested or who have come up negative with current tests.[5]

Widely accepted categories of people may not be useful for estimating the prevalence of HIV infection. Sexual identity does not accurately predict sexual behavior because many self-identified heterosexual men and women, lesbians, and gay men engage in "cross-over" relationships (Goldstein 1995; Scheper-Hughes 1994). Categories of those most at risk, such as needle-sharing drug users and their sexual partners, are usually summations of individual cases; they do not provide data on the community institutions and social networks that can encourage or discourage risk behaviors (Crystal and Jackson 1992; Kane and Mason 1992; Neaigus et al. 1994; Trotter et al. 1996). Familiar groupings, such as "prostitutes," cover a heterogeneous range of women, men, and children who sell a variety of sexual services (Patton 1994). The term blurs important risk variables, such as identity as a professional sex worker, which is more likely to encourage condom use than an ambiguously romantic sexual encounter or bartering sex for drugs.[6] Children who sell sex are the most vulnerable of all, for they are unlikely to make any demands on their customers and often suffer vaginal and anal tears that make HIV infection probable. Particularly vulnerable are poor young women and street children recruited to the sex industry in Latin America and Southeast Asia (Bond 1992; Reid 1990; Wawer et al. 1996).

In sum, the statistics on the prevalence of HIV and AIDS and the social paths of transmission show that they are deeply embedded in social networks and in gendered relationships. Therefore, to understand what the statistics mean for the people affected and their families and what health care and public health policies should be built on them, one must look at the social contexts of risk.

Social Paths of Transmission

Everyone is not at the same risk for AIDS. The transmission of HIV infection clusters by race, class, gender, sexual behavior, intravenous drug use, and access to medical treatment for other sexually transmitted diseases (Altman 1994; Gagnon 1992; Schneider 1992). These social factors produce the overall risk of exposure to HIV infection. Physiological vulnerability to becoming infected also varies; not everyone who is exposed becomes HIV positive or rapidly develops AIDS symptoms. The discovery in 1996 of a genetic mutation that prevents the virus from locking onto cells means that a considerable number of people throughout the world have a built-in protection against HIV infection and an even larger number a delay in breakdown of their immune systems.[7] According to the early reports, the CKR5 mutation is found only in Caucasian people and in a small percentage of those who were exposed but not infected (Dean et al. 1996; Liu et al. 1996; Samson et al. 1996). The search for other genes for immunity or resistance in other populations is proceeding.

Epidemiologists now talk of Pattern I and Pattern II countries, with different types of HIV transmission profiles and core groups—"small numbers of highly sexually active individuals with large numbers of partners who mix with individuals who would otherwise be deemed at a low risk of infection" (Bloor 1995:16). Pattern I countries are in the developed or Westernized world: The main sources of transmission are unprotected anal intercourse and use of unsterile equipment to inject drugs; most of those with HIV infection or AIDS are men; the core groups are (a) promiscuous men who have unprotected sex with men and (b) men and women drug users who share needles and syringes. Pattern II countries are in the developing part of the world, mainly Africa, Asia, and India: The main source of transmission is heterosexual intercourse; almost half of those with HIV infection or AIDS are women; the core groups are (a) women who sell or barter sexual services and (b) migrant men workers, such as truck drivers and workers who leave their wives to run the family farm while they seek employment in the city (Bloor 1995). The likelihood of a generalized heterosexual epidemic of AIDS in the developed world is still open to debate (Bloor 1995:53-54).[8]

Among white middle-class men in the United States, transmission of the virus that causes AIDS is usually through unprotected anal penetration; among poor Black men, the prime risk is from contaminated needles and syringes during injection drug use. For poor Black women and Latinas, the danger is injection drug use and sleeping with men who inject drugs; middle-class women are the most vulnerable when their partners are bisexual, hemophiliacs, or injection drug users (Chu and Wortley 1995; Lewis 1995; Rosenblum et al. 1993; Schneider 1992; Stokes et al. 1996).[9] Cindy Patton (1994) sums up the range of transmission risks: "The clearest and most accurate ranking of probable routes of transmission . . . [is] needle sharers at highest risk, followed by receptive partners in intercourse, regardless of gender" (p. 103).[10] However, men are more likely to share needles than women, and women are, with gay men, those who are penetrated. The powerlessness of the penetrated is the essence of vulnerability to HIV infection.

The Gender Politics of Risk

In Mexico, Brazil, and in the Asian sex tourism industry, gender and sexual categories are overridden by relationships of power and dominance. Men who define themselves as heterosexual engage in anal penetration of men and women lovers, male and female sex workers (who are often very young), and their own wives (Alonso and Koreck 1989; Bloor 1995; Parker 1992). Nancy Scheper-Hughes (1994), an anthropologist who has done extensive fieldwork in Brazil, blames

> the special place of a liberated sexuality in the Brazilian male social imaginary, as an imagined space where everything is permitted, nothing is forbidden, and where sexual sin does not exit. [Anthropologists] note the "catholicity" of sexual tastes and preferences within the Brazilian sexual ideology: for anal/oral sex across all sexual identities; for inter-racial and inter-generational sex; and above all, a fluid and pervasive bisexuality. (p. 993)

The range of sexual behaviors and not sexual identifications together with gender differences in social power should be kept in mind in any discussion of HIV risk factors.

To a great extent, the risks of sexual transmission depend not so much on individual sexual behavior but on sexual *relationships*. Condoms are widely known to be the best protection against HIV infection as well as other sexually transmitted diseases.[11] But condoms are infrequently used in long-term heterosexual or homosexual relationships because "condom use may be perceived as signaling a lack of trust in one's partner and because a partner toward whom one has affectionate feelings is usually not perceived as a potential source of the disease, regardless of the risk history of the individual" (Kelly 1995a:346). As one young woman said, "We've entered a period where mistrust equals responsibility, where fear signifies health" (Daum 1996:33). Whatever the gender composition, the closer the relationship, the less likely the partners are to practice safe sex.

Men and Women

As of 1992, the chief route of transmission of HIV for women in the United States is unprotected heterosexual intercourse with infected partners. The rates are higher among Black women and Latinas than among white women because they are more likely to live in poor communities with a high incidence of drug use, violence, rape, commercial sex, and multiple partners (Hammonds 1992; Lewis 1995; Nyamathi and Vasquez 1989). Women sex workers were accused of spreading the disease (Campbell 1991; King 1990), but then came reports that a woman is much more vulnerable to HIV infection from intercourse with an HIV-positive man than a man is from an HIV-positive woman—ejaculate is an excellent conveyer of the virus, and semen stays in the vagina for days (Nicolosi et al. 1994; Padian et al. 1987, 1991).[12] A study of 379 monogamous heterosexual white couples in their 30s who were followed over five years found that only 1 of the 72 men whose woman partners were HIV positive became infected, whereas 20 percent of the 307 women with HIV-positive male partners did (Padian et al. 1991).

Because of the rising incidence of HIV infection among heterosexual women, the World Health Organization has called for the development of a vaginal microbicide, a virus-killing cream or foam whose use would not depend on the cooperation of men partners (L. Altman 1993). In a speech delivered at the 1996 International AIDS Conference, Donna E. Shalala, U.S. Secretary of Health and Human Services, said that the National Institutes of Health and the Centers for Disease Control and Prevention would spend $100 million to develop such an alternative to condoms and the yet-to-be-developed vaccines by the year 2000 (Altman 1996d). The reason for the concerted effort to develop microbicides is that it is now recognized that women need protection that is under *their* control during sexual intercourse. Safer sex for men is in their hands, literally, if they use condoms. But women find it very difficult to get their men sexual partners to use condoms if they don't want to (Wermuth, Ham, and Robbins 1992). Women have feared violent reactions to their insistence on condom use and to getting tested for the virus (Cooper 1995:287).

Ironically, it is harder for women to insist on condom use or safer sex practices in love relationships than in casual encounters or when partners are paying for sex. In a study of 377 women of varied race and class living in Florida, 74 percent of the 268 with a main partner said they used condoms less than half of the time they had vaginal or anal intercourse, whereas 70 percent of the 109 with client partners reported condom use more than half the time (Osmond et al. 1993). This study also found that when condoms were used it was overwhelmingly because the woman made the decision and her partner agreed to it and that women were more assertive and men more compliant when sex was for sale. However, the African American women in the Florida study were much more successful than the white women or Latinas in getting their main partners to use condoms (86 percent of the time compared to an average for all of 26 percent); they also were in more unstable relationships and less dependent economically on their main partners.

These studies suggest that the success of communication and assertiveness training for women may be more protective in casual sexual encounters than in long-term relationships (DiClemente and Wingood 1995; Sosnowitz 1995). Carole Campbell (1995) criticizes the premises of risk control programs that put the onus on women to learn how to negotiate condom use:

> These strategies serve to reinforce the idea that safer sex is a female concern and responsibility. They fail to address the issue of why women should even have to negotiate safer sex in the first place. That is, they fail to address why safer sex is not a male concern and responsibility. (p. 205)

In recognition of women's relative powerlessness in heterosexual encounters, they are held less accountable than men are for getting AIDS from unprotected consensual sex (Borchert and Rickabaugh 1995).

Despite the recognized difficulty that women have in convincing their male partners to use condoms, the emphasis in Western-oriented prevention programs is on education and individual responsibility. Such programs, argues Scheper-Hughes (1994), "cannot possibly reach that vast unorganized 'non-community' of sexually dominated women for whom the best line of defense might come in the form of widespread and routine testing with follow-up through partner notification" (p. 996). However, unless those men who are infected with HIV are quarantined, as has been done in Cuba, these classic public health measures will not be any more protective of women in long-term heterosexual relationships than lessons in persuasion.

Men and Men

Although many feminists have deplored the powerlessness of women in trying to get male lovers and husbands to use condoms, so that "romantic sex . . . is *unsafe* sex" (Osmond et al. 1993:116), studies of gay men have found the same phenomenon: "Penetrative sex occurs most frequently with a regular sexual partner and, as in heterosexual relationships, is seen as emblematic of intimacy, love and trust; sex with regular partners is much more likely to involve unsafe sex than sex with casual partners" (Bloor 1995:57). Such a division between protected casual sex and unprotected monogamous sex has considerable risk because in both same-gender and cross-gender romantic relationships, there is often overconfidence about a partner's fidelity.

Among gay men in Australia, casual sex with partners picked up in public places is infrequently anal-genital; that sexual practice is more typical of long-term relationships—it conveys trust, intimacy, relatedness, reciprocal give-and-take, and a denial of their own past sexual relationships (Connell and Kippax 1990). The paradox, therefore, is that condoms are least used where they are most needed:

> To the extent that "safe" sex is identified with using condoms for anal sex (a very common understanding), and anal sex is identified with intimacy and relationship, then the less intimate sexuality of the beat [public sexual encounter] may seem not to require precautions. On the other hand, sex in relationship being connected with an ideal of monogamy ("being the only one") may be seen as "safe" *because of the relationship*. Most of the respondents who are currently in couple relationships practice unprotected anal sex with their lovers *whether or not* they are sure their partners have no other sexual contacts. Where the medical definition of prevention conflicts with the social definition of relationships and practices, the social meanings prevail. (Connell, Davis, and Dowsett 1993:123)

Casual sex by men with multiple partners was the original supposed cause of AIDS, before the HIV virus was tracked down. Such sex without attachment is, in Western culture, "hypermasculine sexuality," an adoption of dominant norms by a stigmatized group (Kimmel and Levine 1991). Recognizing the glamour of the "stud," one technique of HIV education has been to use "gay heroes"—locally popular gay men—as educators and safe-sex mentors (Kelly et al. 1991). What is taught, however, tends to be filtered through local beliefs, so that men who routinely and intentionally have unprotected anal and oral sex often justify what they do with reasons based on their own interpretations of public health definitions of risky sexual practices (Levine and Siegel 1992). Others feel fatalistically that becoming infected is inevitable (Gold, Skinner, and Ross 1994).

Women and Women

If men who have sex with men have been the group with the highest risk of becoming HIV positive in the United States, then women who have sex with women should be the group with the lowest risk (Chu and Wortley 1995:5). The rates of female-to-male transmission are low, so the rates of female-to-female transmission should be even lower (Chu et al. 1990). Lesbian-identified women who are injection drug users and who have sexual relationships with men should be at the same risk as heterosexually identified women. There are two problems with this logic. First, no one really knows the transmission risks of lesbian sexual practices, such as oral-genital contact and the shared use of sex toys (Goldstein 1995; Gómez 1995; Kennedy et al. 1995; Patton 1994). Second, women who primarily have sex with women seem to be more at risk when they do have sex with men and when they inject drugs than women who only have heterosexual relationships—they are less likely to use condoms and more likely to exchange sex for crack cocaine and also to have other sexually transmitted diseases (Bevier et al. 1995; Gómez 1995).

Amber Hollibaugh (1995), director of the Lesbian AIDS Project, targets the belief that "true" lesbians don't get AIDS as the source of their possibly greater risk in sexual relationships than female transmission rates would predict. She points out that trust and emotional intimacy are the hallmarks of lesbian relationships: "It is hard to imagine, then, how to begin discussing safer sex, negotiating with a lover, HIV and STD protection methods, talking openly about our drug or sex histories" (p. 228). Yet vaginal yeast infections and sexually transmitted diseases are passed between women lovers. Without accurate knowledge of what sexual behaviors are dangerous, particularly during menstruation, women who have sex with women *are* at risk: "Lesbianism is not a condom for AIDS" (p. 230).

The Politics of Prevention

A 1988 public health campaign in Australia, called "Beds," showed a couple in bed surrounded by other couples in other beds—raising questions about "how many partners they have had, how many partners their partners had had, and so on, developing an exponential vision of a society in which the chain of HIV infection stretched far and wide" (Lupton, McCarthy, and Chapman 1995:100). But despite the recognition that one's partner is sexually experienced, the deeper the relationship, the more the previous history is neither discussed nor acted on.

Even knowledge of a long-term partner's HIV-positive status may not prevent unprotected sex if the alternative is giving up the relationship.

Long-term relationships are embedded in tightly interlocked networks whose norms, based on trust and loyalty, may foster high-risk behavior. As an intensive study in a New York City area with a high incidence of HIV infection found,

> Fully 70% of the drug injectors interviewed . . . injected or shared syringes with a spouse or sex partner, a running partner, or with friends or others whom they knew. . . . [T]he social relationship of drug injectors with members of their risk network were often based on long-standing multiplex relationships, such as those based on kinship, friendship, marital and sexual ties, and economic activity. The intertwining of drug using relationships with these other social relationships implies that attempts to reduce HIV risk behavior among drug injectors may have ramifications for these other relationships, which in turn may either facilitate or hinder the success of such attempts. (Neaigus et al. 1994:75-76)

The way to change sexual behavior may be to foster community norms that "emphasize safer sex as a way for people to show their concern, love, affection, and care for one another" (Kelly 1995a:346).[13] Scheper-Hughes (1994) would likely say that the "commandments" those infected with HIV in Cuba must swear to if they want to live outside confinement in sanitariums are more effective: "To have unprotected sex with an unknowing, uninfected individual is murder. Consensual sex with an uninfected and informed partner is criminal" (p. 999).

Prevention has been more successful in casual sexual behavior. A long-term study of 3,066 women streetwalkers in New York City found a substantial decline in HIV infection in response to an intensive program of distribution of condoms and dental dams, bleach kits, food, and sleeping bags, and counseling and referral to agencies for further help (Whitmore et al. 1996). In his discussion of prostitute women, Michael Bloor (1995) notes that "it is one of the ironies of the HIV epidemic that the public health has been preserved by the efforts of one of the most vilified and marginalized groups in society" (p. 75).

Other programs calling for condom use, fewer sexual partners, safer sex, and abstinence have reduced infection rates. Thailand and Uganda have substantially reduced their heterosexual infection rate through education and low-cost condoms (Altman 1996b). In San Francisco, which has a large population of men who have sex with men, new infections have dropped to 1,000 per year, compared to 8,000 in the early 1980s.[14] But since the late 1980s, there has been discussion of a possible "second wave" of infection among young homosexual men in San Francisco who are fatalistic about the prevalence of AIDS (Bloor 1995; Dunlap 1996b; Gross 1993).[15]

The pervasive stigma suffered by those who are HIV positive and even more, those with AIDS symptoms, may lift if proneness to the infection and the disease are linked to the lack of a genetic mutation entirely beyond the control of the individual.[16] It should change the sense of alienation and almost reverse stigma felt by gay men who are HIV negative, who will now be joined by a blessed group of the genetically endowed (Fisher 1996).[17] The "elect" who have the mutation may be sought after as sexual partners by both the HIV positive and the HIV negative.

To take the responsibility to protect a partner, you have to know whether you are or are not infected and that means getting tested for HIV infection. The fatalism over the inevitability of becoming infected is extended to getting tested. Gender politics also enter the picture, as women may be afraid to reveal their HIV-positive status to an abusive partner. The most controversial issue around testing for HIV is whether it should be mandatory for pregnant women, so that they can take drugs to prevent the transmission of the virus to their newborn infants.

To Test or Not to Test

A politically loaded issue in the United States since the 1980s is mandatory testing and what is done with information on positive HIV status (Bayer, Levine, and Wolf 1986). Identification as a member of a targeted group would be stigmatizing in itself, and public use of test results would be a violation of confidentiality and privacy. These same issues have been present in other epidemics where public health measures were instituted. AIDS has not been treated like other epidemics. Unlike other contagious diseases, such as tuberculosis, mass screening has not been used in the United States or other Western countries.[18] And unlike other sexually transmitted diseases, such as syphilis, there are no public health laws that mandate informing sexual contacts that a former or current partner is infected.[19]

Although public health advocates saw widespread voluntary testing with confidentiality of results as a way of limiting the further spread of HIV infection through changed sexual practices, gay men avoided testing because they feared discrimination, surveillance, and psychological devastation (Siegel et al. 1989).[20] Sexual practices could be altered without knowledge of HIV status. When there was a possibility of prevention of AIDS symptoms with early use of AZT, testing for HIV infection had some purpose. In contrast, people whose sexual partnerships were heterosexual have tended to use the test for reassurance—the "worried well" (Lupton et al. 1995).[21]

The issue of screening target groups and informing sexual contacts is one that involves all men and women now, but in the United States, mandatory testing is limited to blood and semen donors, military personnel, health care personnel, immigrants, some new medical insurance applicants, and federal prisoners. The testing issue that has not been resolved affects only women; it is for maternal-infant (vertical) transmission of the HIV virus (Cooper 1995). As with other maternal antibodies, the antibodies to the HIV virus pass through the placenta during pregnancy. These antibodies are the markers of HIV infection in current tests. Their appearance in newborns means that the birth mother is HIV positive. For children in the United States and in Europe, the overall maternal-infant HIV transmission rate is about 2 per 1,000 births, but the rates for U.S. states vary from none to 6.2 per 1,000 in New York (Chu and Wortley 1995:6-7; European Collaborative Study 1991; Sheon et al. 1996).

From 1987 to 1995, the CDC screened the blood of newborns for HIV antibodies anonymously; these were blinded surveys done at the same time as other mandated testing for neonatal disorders. The results of all but the HIV testing were reported to the parents or legal guardians of the child.[22] The HIV test results were then unlinked from their sources and used for epidemiological tracking and for research (Levine 1993). Through education and counseling, the mother was encouraged to request the results of the HIV test, but further postnatal testing and treatment for herself and the child were entirely voluntary. As of February 1997, New York State hospitals are under a legal mandate to disclose the results of their infant's HIV test to the mother (Sontag 1997). The consequences will affect other states' policies.

Given the relatively low level of transmission (75 percent of babies born to known HIV-infected women do not become infected) and the difficulty of determining which infants are testing positive because of maternal antibodies and which are actually infected with the HIV virus, U.S. government and medical commissions continued to oppose mandatory testing for pregnant women and mother-identified testing of newborns through the early 1990s (Bayer 1995). Tests that can more accurately detect HIV infection in infants a month old have since been developed. In addition, in 1994, zidovudine (AZT) was shown to be effective in reducing the rate of HIV infection in babies from 25 to 8 percent when given to HIV-positive pregnant women prenatally and to their newborns in the first few weeks after birth. Despite subsequent data that question the effectiveness of AZT in preventing mother-child transmission (Steketee et al. 1996), the support for mandatory testing has now grown.[23] At its 1996 annual meeting, the American Medical Association reversed its previous stand and recommended mandatory testing of pregnant women and newborns ("Doctors Back AIDS Test" 1996).

In general, mandatory testing scares people away from services; when HIV counseling and services are widely available and testing is voluntary and strictly confidential, pregnant women of every class and color overwhelmingly consent to testing (Cooper 1995:290-91). An official of the Pediatric AIDS Foundation recommended that testing all pregnant women for HIV become a routine part of standard prenatal care (Ammann 1995). A woman could refuse the test (just as any other test or treatment that is not legally mandated can be refused), but she may not know the test is part of the usual workup; women who do know may forego prenatal care without adequate counseling to assure them they had the right to refuse to be tested (Britton 1995).

Ronald Bayer (1995), long an advocate of protecting the right of consent of mothers, notes that prenatal testing of pregnant women and treating those who are HIV positive for the sake of the fetus is completely unethical. It would also entail a high degree of cooperation: an HIV-infected pregnant woman would have to take five doses of AZT a day for up to 6 months to forestall the 1 in 4 possibility of passing the virus on to her infant (Seals, Hennessey, and Sowell 1996). Although the case for postnatal testing and treatment of HIV-infected newborns seems to make more sense, Bayer notes that the use of preventive drugs in asymptomatic children who may not develop AIDS symptoms for years is also questionable. The central ethical question, however, is whose rights take precedence—the mother's or the child's?

From the perspective of obstetricians and pediatricians at large public hospitals with heavy case loads of very poor women from the worst urban ghettoes, mandatory testing is the only way to identify babies who could benefit from early treatment:

> Most babies born with HIV infection were born to mothers who had become infected by intravenous drug use. They were born in understaffed, overextended obstetrical services of inner city hospitals. The experience of pediatricians serving large numbers of babies with AIDS . . . indicated to them that the majority of infected women chose not to be tested even when counseled about the importance of knowing their own HIV status or that of their babies. (Bayer 1995:300-01)

From the point of view of feminist advocates of women's reproductive rights, it is the mothers who need every legal protection of their privacy and right to make decisions for themselves and their children because the majority of them are Black, Latina, poor, and subject to violence and physical and social abuse (Faden, Geller, and Powers 1992).

Mothers With AIDS

The related ethical, public health, and private dilemma is whether a woman who knows she is HIV positive or who is being treated for AIDS symptoms should deliberately become pregnant, or if she does so accidentally, whether she should have an abortion (Faden et al. 1992; Levine and Dubler 1990; Pies 1995). The incidence of pregnancy in women who are HIV positive or suffering from AIDS is quite high in some communities. A study of the 3,915 women patients with HIV infection who received care in more than 90 clinics, hospitals, and private practices in 11 U.S. cities from 1990 to 1994 found that 14 percent were pregnant when the study began and 5.8 percent became pregnant each subsequent year. Of the original 570 who were HIV positive and pregnant, 47 percent were 15 to 19 years old, and 30 percent were between 20 and 24 (Chu et al. 1996).

The pragmatic answer of many in the medical community has been an unequivocal "no" to becoming pregnant and "yes" to terminating a pregnancy. But feminist ethicists and advocates for women have pointed out that methods that are more effective than condoms in preventing pregnancy, such as diaphragms, intrauterine devices, and oral contraceptives, not only do not protect against transmission of HIV but may make transmission more likely by producing vaginal abrasions and changing vaginal secretions (Duerr and Howe 1995; Hutchison and Shannon 1993). Even spermicides can increase the rate of HIV transmission. Sterilization puts an end to fertility. As for obtaining a clinic abortion, it can be financially or physically difficult in general and even more so for HIV-infected women. Drug-induced abortions must be done early, and, as with hormone-based contraception, the drugs may have detrimental effects on HIV-positive women.

Conversely, pregnancy presents risks if a woman is HIV positive or has symptoms of AIDS (Minkoff 1995). There is some evidence that the immune system may be further weakened and the progression of the disease accelerated. Any AIDS treatment must be continued, but unfortunately, the effects of many of the widely used drugs on pregnant women and the fetus are unknown because pregnant (and potentially pregnant) women were, for a long time, excluded from drug trials (Korvick et al. 1996; McGovern, Davis, and Caschetta 1994). Fortunately, one of the most effective AIDS drugs (AZT, or zidovudine) is protective for the fetus, but its effect on pregnant women has not been determined.[24] Since HIV is known to be transmitted during vaginal birth, caesarean sections have been recommended (Minkoff 1995). Breastfeeding, another means of HIV transmission, is not recommended in developed countries if the mother is HIV positive, but the dangers of unsanitary formula feeding make it necessary in Asia and Africa.

As with all calculations of risk, many elements go into the procreative decisions of HIV-positive women. The likelihood of transmission of the virus is relatively low and can be lowered to under 10 percent with prenatal administration of AZT. Women knowingly have children with higher rates of potentially fatal inheritable diseases. Not all children who are HIV positive immediately develop symptoms of AIDS. There has even been a report of a baby who went from HIV positive to HIV negative by the age of five without drug treatment (Bryson et al. 1995). A child has immense intrinsic value, especially in the communities and cultures that many HIV-positive women live in, including the wives of hemophiliacs (Jason et al. 1990). One study showed that women who live with at least one of their children are less likely to have more children (Pivnick 1991). If a child is removed from the mother's care, she often tries to maintain her motherhood by getting pregnant. The potential father's feelings are an important factor, too (Mbizvo and Bassett 1996). Carol Levine (1993) points out that a woman who is HIV positive and decides to have a baby can be praised as a heroine or criticized for selfishness:

> Many women with chronic diseases—and some who are dying—choose to become pregnant, even at considerable risk to themselves. They are treasured by their families and admired by society for doing so. In contrast, HIV-positive women are considered irresponsible for having babies who may face early death and whose care may be a burden to society. Surely class and ethnicity play a role in these societal responses and judgments. (pp. 116-17)

The most pragmatic question is usually not asked—What is the level of care that mothers with AIDS and their children can expect? What is the level of care for anyone with AIDS?

Care Inside and
Outside the Medical System

In 1995, a combination of three drugs was found to substantially reduce HIV blood levels in those newly infected and in those under treatment for full-blown AIDS (Collier et al. 1996; Danner et al. 1995; Markowitz et al. 1995). The virus may still be present in organs and glands, but the drugs inhibit or stop it from weakening the immune system. However, the virus will probably become resistant to the new protease inhibitors, and then the resistant strains will be the ones transmitted (Borman et al. 1996). The drugs are very expensive, the treatment plan is difficult to follow, and the long-term side effects are unknown (Altman 1996e). The new drugs may be beyond the reach of even middle-class people in the United States, since they can cost a patient between $70,000 and $150,000 a year and may not be covered by insurance plans (Kramer 1996). People in the poor areas of Africa, Asia, India, Latin America, and the Caribbean as well as those in Western countries, who constitute 90 percent of the men and women living with the virus that causes AIDS, are unlikely to be treated at all.[25] This contradiction between potential cures and the aura of the incurability of AIDS has appeared over and over again since 1981, the last time concerning AZT (Altman 1996c, 1996f; Erni 1994).[26]

Class, color, ethnicity, and drug use—all the stigmata of the lives of people with AIDS—also work against them when they seek medical services. Poor women of color often feel they have fallen through the cracks of the U.S. health care system and social service agencies (Seals et al. 1995). Antonia Coello Novello (1995), Surgeon General of the United States, listed their problems in getting decent care: Clinics that are not open during hours they can go, too far from their homes, or up flights of stairs they can't climb; no facilities for child care or for buying food for their children or themselves; fragmented care —children in one place, themselves in another, and partners someplace else; language barriers; and cultural insensitivity (p. xii). It is no wonder then that AIDS survival rates have been worse for women than for men in the United States: They come into the medical system later and are poorer, have fewer social supports, have been heavy drug users, and are often homeless and raped and beaten (Melnick et al. 1994). They then receive fragmented care that neither recognizes their particular physical symptoms nor their psychosocial needs (Selwyn, O'Connor, and Schottenfeld 1995).

Patricia Kelly (1995) lays out a blueprint for a clinic for HIV-positive women that would provide "culturally sensitive, women-centered health care that encompasses medical and psychosocial services, prevention, and education" (p. 279). It is a model of care for anyone with a chronic disease that affects their whole life. For comprehensive service, the clinic would have to provide directly or through a simple referral process "HIV testing and counseling, medical care, nursing, psychiatry, social work/case management, health education, and substance abuse treatment" (p. 279). The medical care would have to be general and gynecological as well as specific to AIDS symptoms. Drug treatment programs to help patients become drug free are vital. She recommends pharmacy services, free condoms, nutrition counseling, and child care (or at least a play area). Especially helpful would be a variety of support groups for different types of patients, co-led by a skilled facilitator and a member of the group. Education, counseling, and testing for new patients, their partners, and their children is another set of services the clinic should provide. Kelly (1995) also recommends that such clinics become sites for new drug testing in order to expand their availability to the women who are the largest target population.

All patients—women, men, and children—could use such comprehensive care; when such services are earmarked only for those who are HIV infected, some professionals feel that other patients lose out, and efforts to prevent the spread of HIV infection to the general population are neglected (Rodriguez-Trias and Marte 1995). Also, since many people fear stigma or discrimination on disclosure of HIV or AIDS status, they may be reluctant to use a dedicated clinic (Moneyham et al. 1996).

Because they feel it doesn't meet their needs, some AIDS patients opt out of the medical system altogether, and others use alternative healers and self-administrated alternative medicines while following an intensive drug regimen (Anderson et al. 1993; Kassler, Blanc, and Greenblatt 1991; Sowell et al. 1997). AIDS patients have also obtained experimental drugs through underground networks and pressured governments to speed up testing procedures (Erni 1994).

Most men and women AIDS patients do not have access to comprehensive care, so the support of family and friends is indispensable. Here there is a clear gender, race, and class difference for the populations most at risk. Data from the 1985 and 1987 San Francisco Men's Health Study, where the population was mostly white, single, gay men between the ages of 25 and 54, showed that friends and the community of other openly gay men provided the most social and emotional support—families were more unreliable (Turner, Hays, and Coates 1993). Since these men were all under stress of personal risk and had to care for lovers and friends who were seriously ill and then organize their funerals, the extent of mutual support was extraordinary.

When family members care for kin with AIDS symptoms, they need a support system themselves to deal with their denial, anger, depression, and visions of their loved one already in the grave (Sosnowitz and Kovacs 1992). The families of the poor women of color who constitute the majority of women with AIDS are particularly hard hit. Many of them are headed by single mothers who have just finished caring for their own children when they take on the care of their sick daughters and often equally sick grandchildren (Simpson and Williams 1993). Along with providing physical care and emotional support, most must do battle with government and social service agencies to become legal foster parents, for if they care for their grandchildren informally, they lose out on benefits:

> The social circumstances of most potential kinship foster parents often reflect those of the HIV-exposed children—that is, primarily low-income with few assets or resources. For this group, the problems lie . . . in their inability to finance the immediate needs of the newly extended family. The extraordinary

and cumulative transitional costs may include the expense of relocating to accommodate and support the surviving children; funeral and burial fees for the deceased parent; probate fees to obtain legal guardianship of each child; and delays of two or three months in the transfer of welfare benefits from the deceased mother to the new parent. In fact, many kinship foster parents experience a lengthy financial crisis as a direct consequence of their child-care commitment. (Simpson and Williams 1993:207)

AIDS has been a horrendous disease for professionals as well as lay caretakers on the "front lines." In the first decade (1981-1991), the problems of health care workers were in the forefront as they faced fears of infection and burnout in meeting the overwhelming needs of very sick patients who were often their own age (Horsman and Sheeran 1995, Navarro 1991). In interviews with 26 physicians in Arizona who cared for at least three AIDS patients, Rose Weitz (1992) found that the gay and bisexual doctors were the most stressed by the emotional costs.

A study of the willingness of physicians-in-training to treat people with AIDS surveyed 383 women and men when they were fourth-year medical students and again, three years later, when they had completed most of their residencies (Yedidia, Berry, and Barr 1996). The students attended three medical schools in the New York City metropolitan area and three elsewhere in New York State; 37 percent did their residencies in hospitals in the New York City area, 20 percent in other New York State hospitals, and 43 percent throughout the United States. Their exposure to AIDS patients thus varied. The study found that the factors that increased willingness to treat people with AIDS were faculty encouragement of tolerance and junior physicians' input into training and their own feelings that they could learn from the experience. Students who persisted in expressing negative attitudes toward such patients were clearly homophobic, disgusted by intravenous drug users, and cynical about the value of patient care. The only significant demographic characteristic was gender: Women trainees were not only more willing than men trainees to treat people with AIDS following graduation from medical school, but those who were unwilling at that time were more likely than the reluctant men students to change their minds and become more positive toward AIDS patients.

Nurses, mostly women but increasingly men, too, have been bedside caregivers and managers of care of AIDS patients in clinics and hospitals, in hospices and homes, and in outreach and public health programs (Fraser and Jones 1995). When the emphasis has been on empathic patient-centered care, gay male nurses, lesbians, and recovered alcoholics and drug users have been sought as health care providers. The negative side of this policy is that it makes it almost impossible to get workers' compensation in the event of becoming infected with HIV on the job: "If a nurse belongs to any of the recognized 'risk groups' for HIV and is infected on the job, the chances of being recognized and compensated for an occupational exposure are practically nil" (Fraser and Jones 1995:292).

Many people would think that the worst thing about being a nurse during the AIDS epidemic is seeing so many people die. But when asked what keeps nurses who care for AIDS patients putting up with "low status, long hours, physically demanding work, and oceans of diarrhea," Marcy Fraser and Diane Jones (1995), who have 10 years' experience nursing in the HIV/AIDS program at San Francisco General Hospital, say,

> Nursing people with AIDS is about mortality. The nearness to dying and loss, the mystery of the last heartbeat between life and death attracts us. We prepare patients as best we can for the transition, and we wait. Bearing witness to the very powerful moment of death and sharing those mysteries keeps many of us working in this field. It is an honor and a privilege not lost on AIDS nurses. (pp. 294-95)

In the absence of treatment that could delay the start of AIDS symptoms or lessen their devastating physical and mental effects, learning that you were HIV positive was like going on Death Row. You might not die for years, but you were already sentenced to death. Even without symptoms, you were in a stigmatized status that called for a change in sexual practices and relationships, in self-identity, and in self-worth.[27] You became a member of the category of "lifetime pariahs—the future ill" (Sontag 1990:121-22).

Now that a combination of drugs has actually reversed the progress of AIDS symptoms, restoring patients to where they can work and take care of their families, it appears that AIDS may be turning from a terminal illness into a chronic but manageable disease (Dunlap 1996d, 1996e; Sullivan 1996).[28] If the promise of the protease inhibitors is sustained, then AIDS will more resemble the HIV-positive stage, albeit with the constant danger of opportunistic infections, than the AIDS stage, with its dreaded, calamitous, downhill physical and mental deterioration and inevitable early death.

I would predict that even if (when?) AIDS is "conquered" —becomes a manageable disease instead of a sentence to a horrible death—it will not be socially or culturally neutralized. AIDS has entered the world's mental landscape, and we can't get away from it.

"AIDS Is Everyone's Trojan Horse"[29]

AIDS as a social metaphor for the fragility of bodies and national boundaries has replaced the old plagues—cholera, tuberculosis, and typhus. "The AIDS crisis is evidence of a world in which nothing important is regional, local, limited; in which everything that can circulate does, and every problem is, or is destined to become, worldwide" (Sontag 1990:180). AIDS as the most dreaded disease has replaced cancer, just the way cancer replaced tuberculosis, and tuberculosis replaced leprosy (Sontag 1990). AIDS has changed ideas about sexual behavior and not in ways predicted originally; abstinence, monogamy, and condom use may have been the official recommendations, but innovative sexual practices in all kinds of couplings and social settings have also been the response to the search for "safer sex" (D. Altman 1993). Education programs for teenagers talk about the pleasures of noncoital sexual activities, dubbed "outercourse" (Genuis and Genuis 1996). Most of all, AIDS has transformed the way we think about bodies.

Or, perhaps what has happened is that men now think about their bodies the way women have thought about their bodies—as vulnerable and penetrable. Samuel Delany (1991), in a piece about homosexuals' risk of AIDS, includes a comment from "a concerned and sensitive heterosexual woman friend: . . . 'AIDS has now put gay men in the position that straight women have always been in with sex: any unprotected sexual encounter now always carries with it the possibility of life or death' " (p. 29). The same is true of heterosexual men, some of whom use HIV tests as "a way of re-establishing the integrity of the fragmented and penetrated body, the 'body besieged' in an age in which there are manifold anxieties concerning the purity of bodily fluids and the strength and resilience of one's immune system to fight invasion of viruses such as HIV" (Lupton et al. 1995:104).

For heterosexual women, the heady days of sexual liberation, when the pill and other woman-controlled means of contraception could be relied on, are gone because they don't protect against HIV infection. They never did protect against any other sexually transmitted diseases, but these were, for a while, curable.[30] Even lesbians have begun to worry about their vulnerability now that bisexuality is a familiar part of their sexual vocabularies. Of course, women have never felt as invulnerable as heterosexual men have, for there is always the threat of rape, but for a short while they could feel that they could be sexually adventurous without the fear of unwanted pregnancy.

The descriptions of the takeover of the body's immune system by HIV reflects female body imagery in other ways. HIV is an invader from outside that makes the body physically and socially unclean, contagious, and set apart (Ray 1989). But with retroviruses like HIV, the boundaries between the invader and the body's own cells are blurred. Immune systems protect by producing flexible but specific antibodies tailored to grab onto and neutralize the invasive foreign bodies. HIV, like all retroviruses, gets into the body's immune system cells and alters their DNA so that instead of repelling the virus they replicate it (Abimiku and Gallo 1995). Thus, the defended body gives way to "the semi-permeable self," where it is hard to tell whether the infectious agent comes from within or without (Haraway 1989).

The imagery of a body that becomes "unclean" from within is reminiscent of concepts of menstrual pollution. The imagery of an HIV-infected body with permeable boundaries reflects the physical interchange between pregnant women and fetuses and the emotional interchange between mothers and daughters in psychoanalytic theory.[31]

Even the metaphors that immunologists now use in describing how viruses produce disease have shifted from masculine to feminine imagery. In current descriptions of the human immune system, according to Emily Martin (1994), descriptions of cell "generals" and "soldiers" are being replaced by descriptions of the system as a whole as a vigilant housewife and mother: "The immune system is like your mom that only makes sure that you get good food, eliminates all the bad food, . . . goes about carrying on daily life, the mundane business of feeding and clothing and cleaning its members" (pp. 97, 98).

The human immune system is reactive, flexible, nonlinear, simultaneously subject and object, circular, and constantly in flux (Martin 1994). In neutralizing bacteria and viruses, the body's own cells change, producing the antibodies that signal both the infection and the immune processes. These antibodies then become a permanent protective part of the body. A virus like HIV suppresses this process by locking onto the immune cells, replacing their genetic code with its own and making them into HIV clones. The genetic protection that has been discovered is the absence of a "lock" that the HIV virus needs to get into the immune cells; the protease inhibitors keep the HIV virus from easily bonding with them. In short, the immune system and the virus become parts of one another. These characteristics are resonant of feminist writings on the female body—the sex which is not one but which is open to and flows into the other (Irigaray [1977] 1985).

Thus, AIDS and immunology have transformed the body from a masculinized machine to a feminized integral part of a social and physical environment:

> The contrast between a rigid structure, its parts held in place in an inflexible way, and a loose structure, its parts able to move and change flexibly, is often taken to go along with a contrast between hostility and combativeness on the one hand, and harmony and peace, on the other. (Martin 1994:147)

But this flexibility is not without costs, which are also familiar elements of women's status. In its responsible reflexivity, Martin (1994) says, the immune system presents a series of paradoxes: It is "responsible for everything and powerless at the same time, a kind of empowered powerlessness" (p. 122). There is "tension between the highly desirable side of flexibility—activity, innovation—and the less desirable side—passivity, acquiescence" (p. 146).

In the new imagery, men's and women's bodies are not just passive recipients to be acted on; they are "both objects and agents of practice" (Connell 1995:61). Socialized bodies, through sexual behavior and injected drug use, spread AIDS, and the people who "own" those bodies have been morally blamed and stigmatized for their risky behavior (Lupton 1993). But the body-social link is more complex—viruses become part of the body, living in it for years, sometimes without the "owner" knowing it, in benignly symbiotic or malignantly parasitic relationships. Disease is not an invasion by a foreign element but part of a feedback loop system. The behavior of the social self who, through daily actions, interacts with other bodies and social selves, continuously reconstructs that body, which then acts on the social self. "Through body-reflexive practices, more than individual lives are formed: a social world is formed" (Connell 1995:64). It is this transformation of our social world by AIDS that will always be with us.

Summary

AIDS is a heterosexually and homosexually transmitted disease, and it is also exchanged along with needles among friends and lovers who are intravenous drug users. HIV is also transmitted during childbirth and breastfeeding, turning normal mothering into a risky endeavor for HIV-positive women. One population almost completely HIV infected are hemophiliacs, who were given contaminated blood transfusions in many countries even after there were good methods of sterilization. Many of those afflicted, primarily men, married and unknowingly passed the virus to their wives and children.

The AIDS epidemic is talked of as "exceptional" and has been treated as a "special case" in public health (Scheper-Hughes 1994). In actuality, though, AIDS is not an exception—the problems of this epidemic are the problems of Western and non-Western health care systems writ large, with the same issues of gender, race, and class that have been discussed throughout this book (Rodriguez-Trias and Marte 1995; Schneider 1992).

In AIDS, as in other diseases, epidemiological data collection has been hampered by outmoded categories of risk groups that concentrate on individual characteristics and neglect the patterns of transmission and prevention in local community networks and peer groups. In the past 15 years, tracking has been of supposed dangerous cases—gay men, prostitutes, and intravenous drug users—neglecting middle-class heterosexual men and women. Governments were slow to finance research and low-cost treatments and prevention programs when the populations at risk were poor people of color or women of any race and class, but they prioritized finding a cure when the problem was found to also affect middle- and upper-class heterosexual men.

The premise of this book has been that all diseases are intertwined with social processes: Different social statuses put people at different risks and vary their access to health care. AIDS is certainly no different in this respect. Another premise has been that the social status of those who are ill is not only an effect of their individual sick role behavior but, to an even greater extent, reflects their society's evaluation of them as people. With AIDS, hemophiliacs and their wives are heroic victims of their governments' refusal to purify the blood with which hemophiliacs injected themselves; injection drug users and their wives are stigmatized as perpetrators of their own physical decline even though a government-issued supply of free clean needles would be a cheap way to prevent transmission of the HIV virus.

Health care in Westernized countries is oriented to cure, not prevention; to individual treatment of specific pathologies as they occur, not to strengthening physical, emotional, and social capacities for living with a chronic or recurrent disease. Poor women and men with AIDS in particular have needed, and not obtained, such holistic care. The social supports that have mitigated the ravages of AIDS for middle-class gay men have been supplied by their lovers, friends, and community-organized services, not by the medical system. In non-Westernized countries where much of the population suffers from malnutrition and other infections, AIDS is an epidemic like the medieval Black Death in Europe—a plague that kills a substantial proportion of young adults.

Certainly, the scientific research effort has paid off—the HIV virus was discovered, and more and more of its immune cell-binding properties have been revealed, including genetic and drug protectors. But much less money and time has been spent on the social aspects of transmission and health care. In retrospect, it seems astounding that no one tried to prevent the inevitable spread to injection drug users by contaminated needles, given the scrupulous disposal of needles in medical settings. The assumption that women could not get AIDS unless they were prostitutes is attributable to the moral contrast of categories of people (gay men vs. heterosexual men; prostitute women vs. good women), an astonishingly naive misunderstanding of sexual behavior and sexual practices. Equally naive has been the assumption that education in safe sex and condom use would halt the spread of AIDS in *any* population. Again, the gender dynamics of relationships were ignored, as were the cultural meanings of condoms and social meanings of love and trust.

AIDS has been different from other epidemics in one major respect: Despite dire predictions of quarantine and other means of social control of those who test HIV positive, it has not, at least in democracies, resulted in mandatory testing, increased government surveillance, or loss of civil liberties:

> Out of the controversies that whirled about the antibody test, there emerged a broad voluntarist consensus. Except for clearly defined circumstances, testing was to be done under conditions of voluntary, informed consent, and the results were to be protected by stringent confidentiality safeguards. To underscore the importance of protecting the privacy of tested individuals, the option of anonymity was made broadly available. This consensus was supported by gay leaders, civil libertarians, bioethicists, public health officials, and professional organizations representing clinicians. (Bayer 1995:297)[32]

The downside of this policy of voluntary action is that the onus for protection is placed on the individual, who must be aware of risks and suspicious of sexual partners and constantly negotiate self-protection (Lupton 1993). Into this negotiation go differences in power and privileges, and a gender analysis tells us who usually wins and who usually loses. As Scheper-Hughes (1994) says,

> Until all people—women and children in particular—share equal rights in social and sexual citizenship, an AIDS program built exclusively on individual rights to bodily autonomy and privacy cannot possibly represent the needs of groups who have been historically excluded from these. (p. 1002)

The "strong and humane public health system" she calls for needs to be matched by a medical system sensitive to gender dynamics and gender politics. At the same time, individuals do have to know how to protect their own health *and* the health of those in their intimate networks *and* the health of their children, but they should not be blamed if their immune systems are so weakened by a virus and social and environmental bodily assaults that they ultimately break down.[33] The intricate interplay of individual freedom and institutional protections, of medical care and social needs, of attention to special cases and evenhanded distribution of personal and societal resources —these ambiguities and complexities are the heart of the social construction of all illnesses, and they affect all people, regardless of race, class, sexual orientation, or gender.

Notes

1. Corea 1992; Nechas and Foley 1994; Patton 1994; Rodriguez-Trias and Marte 1995; and Wright et al. 1987.

2. Men who didn't have CDC-designated symptoms were also denied benefits (Crystal and Jackson 1992).

3. On issues in the constructionist perspective on AIDS, see Levine 1992 and Treichler 1988, 1992.

4. The first reports were of pneumocystis carinii pneumonia and Karposi's sarcoma, which produces lesions in the skin, mucous membranes, and internal organs. They are opportunistic infections that affect those with weakened immune systems. They were rarely seen by American physicians before the late 1970s. There are now more than 30 different conditions known to proliferate when immune systems are weakened by HIV.

5. On the discrepancy between data from the Centers for Disease Control, which depends on medical reports, and data from the General Social Surveys, which has asked people how many people they know with HIV infection and AIDS, see Laumann, Gagnon, and Michaels 1993.

6. Since there is a double economy of sex and drugs, the Centers for Disease Control now has the category "people who trade sex for drugs or money" (Patton 1994:56).

7. A double copy of the gene protects against infection; a single copy seems to delay the development of AIDS symptoms by 5 to 10 years.

8. On similarities of migration in developed and developing countries and the potential spread of HIV infection, see Patton 1994, 21-47. For a view that the risk among women has been exaggerated, see Mertz, Sushinsky, and Schuklenk 1996. They claim that the only women truly at risk are those who inject drugs, are ill with other diseases, are poor, and are malnourished.

9. Epidemiologists distinguish three categories of transmission: *primary,* or direct from contaminated needles or blood transfusions or semen and male-to-male sexual contact; *secondary,* from sexual contact with those with primary infections; and *tertiary,* from sexual contact with those with secondary infections.

10. Oral receptive intercourse (fellatio) without a condom or dental dam should be included here as high-risk sexual behavior (Wallace et al. 1992, 1996).

11. "Protection" formerly meant condom use to prevent pregnancy. With the widespread use of the pill and the IUD, condoms have become associated primarily with protection from sexually transmitted diseases. On the varying meanings of condoms in the United States, see Gamson 1990.

12. There has been no way to remove HIV from semen. In artificial insemination, donors must be screened before donation, the semen frozen, and donors retested 6 months later to ensure that they were not infected at the time of donation but before antibodies could be detected (Guinan 1995).

13. Also see Browne and Minichiello 1996; Kelly 1995b; and Lear 1995.

14. Epidemics also stabilize when the population at risk is "saturated"—there are few uninfected people (Bloor 1995:31-32).

15. On the failures of public health campaigns in this population, see Green 1996.

16. At the 8th International Conference on AIDS in 1992, the anomalies of HIV infection were openly discussed (Martin 1994). These were HIV infection without development of AIDS even after 15 years and AIDS-like symptoms in those HIV negative. Some researchers invoked risk-prone versus protective lifestyles as explanations for the differential effects of HIV infection, questioning whether the virus was the sole or sufficient cause of AIDS. A 1995 review of theories about long-term survivors suggested that there might be a mutant HIV strain (Altman 1995a).

17. For a discussion of new concepts of the "fittest," see Martin 1994.

18. The dual epidemics of TB and AIDS has again raised questions of mandatory screening and mandatory and monitored treatment (Bayer, Dubler, and Landesman 1993).

19. See Scheper-Hughes (1994) for a criticism of these policies. For the perspective of a public health official, see Steven Joseph (1992), New York City Commissioner of Health from 1986 to 1990.

20. Weitz's (1992) interviews with physicians in a state with mandatory reporting of positive results of HIV tests showed that they discouraged patients from getting tested, preferring to treat symptoms as they occurred.

21. In the United States, home testing kits went on the market at the end of 1996 (Canedy 1996).

22. Mandated and reportable testing is done for PKU, syphilis, and other congenital disorders. When an infant tests positive for syphilis, it means the mother has it (Bayer 1995).

23. For discussion of these issues, see Bayer 1994, 1995, 1996; Berger, Rosner, and Farnsworth 1996; Connor et al. 1994; and Rogers, Mofenson, and Moseley 1995.

24. On the contradictions of leaving women out of the original AZT trials because the drug might do fetal damage and then designing a trial (ACTG 076) to ascertain how protective of fetuses AZT is, see Corea 1992. ACTG 076 did not monitor the effects of AZT on the pregnant *woman.*

25. The official theme of the 1996 International Conference on AIDS in Vancouver was "One World—One Hope." Alternate slogans going around among the participants were "Third World—No Hope," "New Hope for the Rich," and "Greed-Death" (Dunlap 1996a).

26. What was remarked on as different in 1996 was that the participants in the drug trials included women and were also racially varied (Altman 1996e).

27. Jaccard, Wilson, and Radecki 1995; Massad et al. 1995; Moneyham et al. 1996; Sherr 1995; Tewksbury 1995; and Weitz 1992.

28. A macabre marker of this change in status in the United States is that AIDS patients who want to sell off their life insurance policies to get up-front money for living expenses and medical bills are now finding no takers (Dunlap 1996c). The transactions are known as viatical settlements; for the past 10 years, there has been a thriving financial industry of companies who buy policies at about 65 percent of their face value, expecting a 100 percent death benefit when the original policy-holder dies—the sooner the better.

29. Sontag 1990:168.

30. Gonorrhea soon became resistant to penicillin; the genital and oral herpes viruses are never completely eradicated. These and other sexually transmitted diseases have become almost incurable opportunistic infections in women with AIDS.

31. Haraway (1989) discusses why the pregnant woman does not reject the fetus as a foreign body in note 8, pp. 39-40. For mother-daughter ego boundaries, see Chodorow 1978.

32. For a review of the predictions, see Ray 1989.

33. See Martin (1994) for a discussion of immune system resistance and breakdown. As she indicates, throughout the past 15 years there has been a battle among AIDS researchers between those who have focused on the molecular biology of HIV and those who have focused on host resistance.

CHAPTER 6

Treating Social Bodies in Social Worlds

Feminist Health Care

> In these exchanges the social certainly interrupts and interpenetrates the
> medical. Whether medical or social topics are being discussed,
> social/ideological assumptions are clearly embedded in the discourse.
> (Fisher 1995:59)

I have argued in this book that the human experiences of physical illnesses are
socially constructed and that women's and men's experiences are often quite
different. These differences are not primarily based in biology or physiology.
Although female and male hormones, skeletal structure, and procreative organs
are distinctive, most of the phenomena discussed in this book result from *gender*,
a social status, and not sex, a biological category. Gender differences, like the
racial, ethnic, and class differences that cross-cut them, are the result of *social
factors*, such as economic resources, nutrition, type of work done, family responsibilities, and socioemotional supports. These social factors are embedded in
systems of roles and practices legitimated by norms and values, which sociologists call *institutions*—the economy, the family, the medical system, and the
gender order.

In modern society, *organizations*, such as hospitals, link individuals to institutions (and institutions to each other). A patient in a hospital may be getting sick
pay from a paid work position and medical insurance from a health care agency,
linking the economic and medical systems. The patient is also a family member,
and his or her relationships with spouse, children, siblings, and parents intertwine the medical system with the family as a social institution.

What this book has stressed is that institutions and organizations and their
roles, practices, and values are not neutral but are imbued with gender, race,
ethnicity, and social class. In real life, these statuses have a combined effect, but
researchers try to look at each separately. If exact matches could be found, one
could compare the medical response to patients who differ only on gender: a man
and a woman, both African American, middle-class, 50-year-old divorced bank
managers with cardiovascular problems. The man's irregular heartbeat and
fainting spells would probably elicit a battery of tests and specific treatment; the
woman's identical symptoms would probably elicit a prescription for tran-

quilizers for emotional stress. One could similarly compare the experiences in an infertility clinic of a woman and man who are both white, working-class, 23-year-old married postal clerks with infertility due to adolescent bouts of gonorrhea. The woman may find that her sexual past creates skepticism about her mothering capabilities in the eyes of the staff of the infertility clinic, but the same staff will most probably urge the man's wife to undergo *in vitro* fertilization so he might have a biological child.

Most social research can only approximate such clear-cut comparisons of single variables; for the most part, social science researchers concentrate on the interactive effects of several factors at once. In medical research, though, social factors are often studied separately from the physical processes, if they are studied at all. Because the knowledge base of modern medicine is rooted in the sciences (biology, biochemistry, physiology, endocrinology, and so on), the social and environmental aspects of disease and the experience of illness are given little attention in medical training and practice. The body is dissected in medical school, and its functions and dysfunctions are memorized. But in order to understand the complexities of illness as a social experience, you cannot look only at the patient's body. Even adding emotional reactions is not enough. Illness takes place within a web of interaction that ties together the person concerned, family, friends, coworkers, health care professionals, medical bureaucracies, the physical setting, the technology, government policies and politics, economics, values, knowledge, and beliefs (Brown 1995; Pescosolido 1992).

In teaching medical sociology, I developed a project that I used over the years to help students understand the combined impact of patients' social characteristics on illness careers, sick roles, and encounters with the health care system. This project asked students to analyze the experience of being a patient, using their own experiences or interviewing someone they knew well. They were to ask the following questions:

- What is your age, gender, ethnicity, religion, education, occupation? What is your marital status? How many children or adults are you responsible for? Who do you live with? What effect did any of these social factors have on your getting sick or having an acute episode of a chronic illness?

- What were the initial stages of your illness career in a new illness or a recent acute episode of a chronic illness? What were the symptoms? How did you interpret them? What was the input of other laypeople (family, friends, co-workers, etc.)? What self-medication did you use? At what point and why did you consult a professional in person or by phone? What kind of professional? Why did you choose this professional?

- What was this professional's interpretation of the symptoms? What was the diagnosis? What were the recommendations for treatment? What was your response to this diagnosis and treatment regimen?

- If other physicians or health care workers (e.g., specialists, physical therapists) were consulted, what was their interpretation of the symptoms, their diagnosis, their treatment plan, and how did you respond?

■ Describe what happened in one particular encounter in this illness. What was the setting—for example, general practitioner's office, specialist's office, hospital, emergency room? Who, besides you, was present (professionals, other health care workers, family members)? What were the occupational status and the social characteristics (approximate age, gender, ethnic group, etc.) of the medical staff or other health care workers present? What exactly went on? How was the work divided? Were there areas of conflict or argument? What were they? How were they resolved? How did you feel (satisfied, angry, upset) during and after this medical encounter?

■ Do you think you conformed or deviated from sick role norms throughout this illness (or are conforming or deviating if it is a chronic illness)? Did you comply with the physician's recommendations? Culturally and ethnically, how did your family and friends expect you to behave in the sick role? How did you actually behave in the sick role? What was the response of the others in the situation (laypeople and professionals) to your behavior?

■ How did (or does) the illness impact on your family and work roles? Did you return to normal functioning, or were your occupational and familial status changed by the illness? In what ways did your work and family roles change?

■ Did you become a "permanent patient"? What is your life like?

As you can see, a patient's whole social world is involved in a major illness, and a whole medical world influences one encounter with a health care professional. Although the patient may challenge, resist, and counteract, the assumptions that prevail are likely to be those of the health care professional, especially if she or he is a physician. One way of equalizing the power differential somewhat is for laypeople to become more knowledgeable about medicine and science in general and particularly about any serious illness they may have. Thanks to the consumer movement and the feminist movement, laypeople have become more aware of tests, medications, the causes of different illnesses, treatment alternatives, and likely outcomes. However, what one learns from the mass media has been filtered through several editing processes. First, data produced by researchers in laboratories and clinical trials become part of scientific communications by getting published in professional science and medical journals. To get published, they must conform to certain editorial guidelines. Science reporters then use only the most newsworthy items in the professional publications for their articles in mass media newspapers and magazines and reports on television. Their stories may be the layperson's only source of scientific and medical information, and much that is important is often just not there.

For example, the first reports of double-blind drug trials for AIDS patients using the new protease inhibitors appeared in medical journals at the end of 1995 (Markowitz et al. 1995). They were brought to the attention of the wider medical and science communities early in 1996 (Cohen 1996; Mellors 1996). At the time of the Vancouver International Conference on AIDS in July 1996, *The New York Times* called the combined treatment of new and older drugs a "medical watershed" in a front-page story (Altman 1996e). A background story (Dunlap 1996a) and a summary in the science section (Altman 1996f) shaped the account into a narrative. This "story" gave hope that AIDS might soon become a manageable, chronic, but not inevitably fatal disease, and even be cured completely. However, a cautioning Op-Ed page commentary (Rotello 1996) told a different story, warning that the virus would probably develop resistance to the protease inhibitors as it had to other drugs and would probably continue to lurk in tissues or the brain. When transmitted, it would be harder to cure. The "story" about resistance had also appeared in a medical journal (Borman, Paulous, and Clavel 1996), but it was not as newsworthy and did not make the front page.

In less life-threatening situations, taking a routinely prescribed drug might lead to life-threatening side effects. Postmenopausal women are often given hormone replacement therapy even if they are not bothered by hot flashes, the rationale being that it prevents heart attacks and bone loss. But it may increase the risk of breast cancer. Even the best-informed woman finds it hard to make good choices, especially when there is little discussion in medical and lay media about the need for hormone replacement therapy in the first place. For example, the underlying assumption in a roundtable discussion on international responses to hormone replacement therapy published by the *Journal of Women's Health* was that long-term estrogen replacement therapy was an established medical practice, not to be questioned (Roundtable Discussion 1996). Only 1 of the 10 women physicians from Denmark, Italy, Germany, Canada, and the United States who participated in the roundtable brought up useful alternative treatments. They focused instead on the assessment of different risk factors (bone loss, cardiovascular disease, and breast cancer) and compared insurance costs of routine lifetime estrogen use versus testing and targeted use. The section called "The Patient's Perspective" discussed educating patients, compliance, and national differences in acceptance of lifetime drug use. The patient's reluctance to take hormones for the rest of her life was presented as a problem for the physician, not as a legitimate viewpoint. The roundtable was sponsored by Eli Lilly and Company, one of the largest drug manufacturers of estrogens.

The research reported in this book shows that women and men doctors differ both in attention to women patients' symptoms and recommendations for tests and in communication styles. Although small and subtle, physicians' gender differences combined with racial and ethnic cultural sensitivity may be enough to attract patients of the same gender, race, and ethnic group.[1] These patients hope to get a physician who understands their point of view, but how much the doctor's social characteristics modify their professional training and basic modes of practice is hard to tell. In their biomedical perspective and reliance on drug therapies, there is little difference between women and men physicians.

The demographics of the medical profession are changing, and physicians are likely in the near future to be mostly women of diverse racial and ethnic groups. With the spread of payment by governments or large insurance companies, the authority of doctors has been eroded and their incomes have gone down. At the same time, consumer movements have diminished their prestige. As a result, fewer men are going into medicine, leaving room for more women, who are fast becoming the majority of doctors in every country with a Western medical system. But these women physicians are not challenging medicine's biology-based perspective. Medical school curricula and training are still focused on individual bodies and their pathologies, with a smattering of courses in public health, environmental and occupational diseases, nutrition, stress, and family medicine.

Much medical care is delivered by nonphysician personnel, especially nurses, the majority of whom are women. Yet their numbers have not made the medical profession as a whole a woman-dominated one in practices and values because the professional hierarchy puts physicians at the top of the authority chain. Physicians' power to define the medical encounter comes from their authority as experts in medical science. The values of science are objectivity and emotional distancing (Keller 1985). These values are only partially softened by nursing's ethic of care and concern for the patient. In technology-based medicine, nurses are more often busy with the mechanics and instrumentalities of patient care than with dispensing TLC. Listening to the patient's emotional and social problems is relegated to nurses' aides and other personnel even further down the medical hierarchy. And even they don't get paid to listen; they get paid to do physical care.

The social factors that construct health and illness are, for the most part, bracketed off and ignored in Western medicine. What if they were an integral part of medical knowledge and medical practice? What if the patient's perspective and the caring ethic of nurses were truly integrated into treatment regimens? What if the medical hierarchy were flattened, and the patient or patient's representatives were given complete information in an understandable way and encouraged to take responsibility for all decisions? What if the participants in clinical trials were not only diversified but their experiences were built into the testing protocols? What if funds for research were funneled to find the environmental causes of and solutions for common and devastating health problems and not siphoned off to enhance careers or produce salable drugs?

These proposals have become part of what is sometimes called "feminist health care." Although the original focus was on women's health care needs, the feminist perspective is appropriate for everyone's health care. As Alice Dan (1994) says in her introduction to *Reframing Women's Health,* "Why should context be any more significant for women than for men? Men's lives are also lived within a context" (p. xv). The normative assumptions about health and illness may be built on men's lives and minimize women's special needs, but views of "normality" also ignore the health care needs of working-class men, men of color, and bisexuals and homosexuals. If health care were to be "reframed" along feminist perspectives to everyone's benefit, what would it look like?

Feminist Health Care

Social Bodies and Social Epidemiology

Humans can differ genetically, hormonally, physiologically, environmentally, and socially from prenatal development to death, and much research time and effort has gone into trying to separate out causal factors for a variety of illnesses and pathologies. From a biomedical perspective, isolation of the prime cause (a gene or genetic mutation, a hormone or its lack, an element of diet, exercise, smoking, and so on) is the ideal, modeled after the identification of specific bacteria that cause specific diseases.[2] This century has seen the design of insulin, vitamins, vaccines, and antibacterials to handle diseases caused by specific deficiencies or invaders, but researchers now face chronic disorders of the cardiovascular, respiratory, and immune systems. These diseases are responsive to social factors, such as the way we live and work, and to the environment, which can trigger genetic predispositions. Social epidemiology has also traced the transmission and spread of bacteria and viruses along paths of social interaction and documented the physiological effects of access to prevention and early treatment.

The biological-social interaction is a feedback loop. Bodies affect social life, and social life affects bodies. What bodies are doesn't dictate behavior; people with relationships and social ties and social statuses decide how their bodies should act. Rather than alter risky behavior, we often expect that there will be a medical technology developed to deal with the consequences of our actions—cures for sexually transmitted diseases, orthopedic surgery for sports traumas. But if the body cannot be restored to whatever passes for normal in a particular society, the society can adapt to encompass a range of bodies —as in the Paralympics, where people in wheelchairs race each other, where those with one leg do high jumps, and those who cannot see play games with bell-ringing balls.

In sum, to understand the incidence, prevalence, and transmission of any disease, social epidemiologists have to consider a population's body typologies, social practices that affect bodies directly (what people eat, drink, smoke), social environments (where people live, the work they do), social and sexual networks that influence individual behavior and provide emotional supports, and access to health-care resources, technology, and knowledge. Similarly, a context-based health practice looks at the whole life of an individual to understand the cause and effects of a set of symptoms and to decide on the most productive course of treatment and adaptation to diminished capabilities.

Participatory Medical Encounters

If patients are going to be full participants in medical encounters, they must be given time to describe the context of a particular illness episode and its time span (Candib 1988). In turn, the health care professional must "accept as valid another person's experience in shaping his or her way of looking at the world," and in "listening actively," indicate that she or he respects the patient's interpretation of events surrounding the illness (p. 135). Lucy Candib (1987) goes even further, recommending that when the health care professional shares a similar life experience she should talk about it with a patient who is describing an emotionally disturbing event, such as a child's illness or a parent's death. But she warns that such sharing can put an undue burden on a patient, who may see it as a bid for sympathy or feel coerced to behave the same way the doctor did. It might be better to find a more general area of common identity, as parents of preschoolers or as bike riders, or a common background, such as growing up in a similar neighborhood.

Participatory medical encounters seem to call for an ideal situation—an unhurried professional and a familiar patient. But as all the accounts of medical encounters show, when asked "What's wrong?" patients do say what's bothering them and why it is of concern to them, how long the problem has been going on, and, if given the chance, narrate its history. It's not lack of time to listen that's the difficulty, it's that physicians, in particular, hear only what *they* think is important to know—the cues for the physical, body-located source of the "abnormality." They cut off the patient's story because they rarely credit social factors, such as losing a job, as an equally valid reason for someone getting sick or getting worse. When prescribing remedies, because they have not listened to the context of the individual patient's life, they are likely to stereotype, assuming, for instance, that a disabled woman doesn't want children or that a young woman is sexually active with a man (Haas 1994; Nosek 1992; Nosek et al. 1995).

Sue Fisher (1995) points out that although caring is the hallmark of nursing, and nurse practitioners pride themselves on probing for the social aspects of a patient's symptoms, they, too, are likely to try to impose their definition of the situation as the solution to the patient's overall difficulties. Thus, in a case she analyzes, the nurse practitioner discusses divorce with a patient whose marital difficulties have made her ill, but the patient resists that solution. Since nurse-patient encounters are less asymmetrical in authority and power than those between doctors and patients (especially when the doctor is a man and the patient a woman), there is more room for "bargaining." In Fisher's case, the compromise suggested by the patient and validated by the nurse practitioner is to go out more with her friends and take up running again.

There is no doubt that patients have to struggle to make themselves heard in most medical encounters and that a more open "ear" on the part of practitioners would help reveal the "multilayered, complex, and fluid" aspects of illnesses (Fisher 1994:326). But doctors, nurses, and patients have social identities and viewpoints that may conflict, and the given in any *medical* setting is that the professional has the authority, power, prestige, and greater knowledge. A feminist practice puts the burden of change on the professional, not the patient. It is up to the professional to make sure that he or she hears the patient's description of both the physical symptoms and the social context, that the patient understands the physiological aspects of the problem and the alternatives for treatment (and nontreatment, too), and that the patient makes the decisions (not just agrees to them) and is given support and referrals even if the professional doesn't agree with the decisions.

Social Worlds and Expert Knowledge

Because so many women patients' voices go unheard, some feminists have recommended the development of a specialty in women's health that is not "a reproductive surgical specialty" but, rather, treats women "as whole human beings with minds, bodies, and spirits—separate and distinct from men's—and worthy of an equal investment in scientific study, clinical education, and medical services" (Johnson and Hoffman 1994:36, 37). This specialty would be interdisciplinary, treating lung and colon cancer as well as ovarian cancer and domestic violence and rape as well as infertility. There have been proposals for similar women's health care nurse practitioner programs to provide primary health care addressed to women's needs (Cohen et al. 1994). A women's health medical and nursing specialty would be similar to gerontology, adolescent medicine, and pediatrics, which serve the special physical, psychological, and social problems of people of different ages. It would remedy the fragmentation of care among gynecologists, internists, family practitioners, and other specialists.

An alternative approach to women's health care is to create expert knowledge that could be taught to family practitioners and other primary care physicians. In 1990, under the auspices of the American Medical Women's Association, a group of women representing medical societies and women's health consumer organizations drafted a core curriculum "to improve and integrate the care of women patients, heighten physicians' awareness of the psychosocial aspects of women's treatment, improve the physician-patient partnership, and increase the physicians' understanding of the differences and unique qualities of women's health" (Wallis 1994:21). The curriculum is divided into five life-phase modules (early years, young adult, midlife, mature years, and advanced years) and covers nine content areas: sexuality and reproduction, women and society, health maintenance and wellness, violence and abuse, mental health and substance abuse, transition and changes, patient-physician partnership, normal female physiology, and diagnosis and management of conditions common to the five age groups. Michelle Harrison (1994), who is not in favor of a separate women's health specialty because she feels that all of medicine and health care should address the needs of women, nevertheless suggests a master's degree in women's health, the recipients of which could then develop programs, design research, and teach a variety of health care personnel.

Women's health cannot be divorced from international political and economic structures: "Gender relations, ethnic relations, class relations, and international relations are intertwined in systems that have very efficient self-perpetuating mechanisms" (Barroso 1994). Attention to living and working conditions, adequate food, and prevention of diseases are the foundation of good health for women and men. What is crucial for women is that they are more likely to be poor and powerless.

Feminist men concerned with men's health have pointed out that just as women's overall social status makes them vulnerable to illnesses of poverty and to procreative and sexual coercion, so does men's social status put them at risk for traumas, drug and alcohol abuse, homicide, and suicide (Sabo and Gordon 1995a). Given the gender-segregated structure of work, men's jobs are often physically hazardous. Norms of masculinity shape their responses to traumas: Boys are taught to "play through pain" and also to deny or ignore illness symptoms. Men in middle management suffer the stress of responsibility with too little authority and little encouragement to talk about their feelings. Fathers are discouraged by their employers from taking time to spend with their children, even in countries that mandate paid paternal leave in the first year of a child's life. Poor men, who are most likely to be suffering from multiple physical problems, usually have the most difficulty in obtaining comprehensive care. These are the social contexts of men's illness that could easily become the focus of a new men's health movement that critiques the gendered social structure: "Men's roles, routines, and relations with others are fixed in the larger historical and structural relations that constitute the gender order" (Sabo and Gordon 1995b:16).

Gender together with race, culture, and social class constitute the grounding for individually experienced pathologies. Women's and men's illness and health are deeply embedded in the *social* order. The expert knowledge for comprehensive health care has to start with *social worlds*—of women and of men of different races, cultures, religions, and economic classes—and work back from social processes to their impact on bodies. In practice, that knowledge can be applied to particular patients, working back and forth from their social worlds to their socially constituted bodies. The knowledge of different social worlds should not be confined to practitioners from those worlds—I am not suggesting that only practitioners who share all a patient's social characteristics can treat that patient. What is more important is that practitioners from different social worlds learn about health and illness through the prism of the social, which refracts the supposedly universal human body and its functions and dysfunctions into diverse and various *social bodies*.

Notes

1. In the United States, religion used to group communities of physicians and patients, but it is less of a factor today than race, ethnicity, and gender.

2. The transmission and spread of these bacteria, however, follow paths of social interaction.

R E F E R E N C E S

Abbey, Antonia, Frank M. Andrews, and Jill L. Halman. 1991. "Gender's Role in Responses to Infertility." *Psychology of Women Quarterly* 15:295-316.

Abimiku, Alash'le G. and Robert C. Gallo. 1995. "HIV: Basic Virology and Pathophysiology." Pp. 13-31 in Minkoff, DeHovitz, and Duerr. New York: Raven Press.

Abplanalp, Judith M. 1983. "Premenstrual Syndrome: A Selective Review." *Women and Health* 8(2-3):107-23.

Allen, Machelle. 1994. "The Dilemma for Women of Color in Clinical Trials." *Journal of the American Medical Women's Association* 49:105-09.

Alonso, Ana Maria and Maria Teresa Koreck. 1989. "Silences: 'Hispanics,' AIDS, and Sexual Practices." *Differences: A Journal of Feminist Cultural Studies* 1(Winter):101-24.

Altman, Dennis. 1993. "AIDS and the Discourses of Sexuality." Pp. 32-48 in *Rethinking Sex: Social Theory and Sexuality Research*, edited by R. W. Connell and G. W. Dowsett. Philadelphia: Temple University Press.

Altman, Lawrence K. 1993. "New Strategy Backed for Fighting AIDS." *The New York Times*, November 2, pp. C1, C3.

———. 1994. "Obstacle-Strewn Road to Rethinking the Numbers on AIDS." *The New York Times*, March 1, p. C3.

———. 1995a. "Long-Term Survivors May Hold Key Clues to Puzzle of AIDS." *The New York Times*, January 24, pp. C1, C11.

———. 1995b. "AIDS Is Now the Leading Killer of Americans from 25 to 44." *The New York Times*, January 31, p. C7.

———. 1996a. "AIDS Meeting: Signs of Hope and Obstacles." *The New York Times*, July 7, Sunday News Section, pp. 1, 8.

———. 1996b. "India Suddenly Leads in HIV, AIDS Meeting Is Told." *The New York Times*, July 8, p. A3.

———. 1996c. "At AIDS Meeting, Experts Find an Uneasy Mix of H" *The New York Times*, July 9, p. C5.

———. 1996d. "AIDS Researchers Differ on Vaccine Strategies." *The Times*, July 10, p. C10.

―――. 1996e. "Scientists Display Substantial Gains in AIDS Treatment." *The New York Times,* July 12, pp. A1, A16.

―――. 1996f. "Discussing Possible AIDS Cure Raises Hope, Anger and Questions: What Exactly Is Meant by 'Cure'?" *The New York Times,* July 16, p. C3.

American Medical Association Council on Ethical and Judicial Affairs. 1991. "Gender Disparities in Clinical Decision Making." *Journal of the American Medical Association* 266:559-62.

Ammann, Arthur J. 1995. "Unrestricted Routine Prenatal HIV Testing: The Standard of Care." *Journal of the American Medical Women's Association* 50:83-84.

Andersen, Arnold E., ed. 1990. *Males with Eating Disorders.* New York: Brunner/Mazel.

Anderson, Elijah. 1989. "Sex Codes and Family Life among Poor Inner-City Youths." *Annals of the American Academy of Political and Social Science* 501:59-78.

Anderson, W., B. B. O'Connor, R. R. MacGregor, and J. S. Schwartz. 1993. "Patient Use and Assessment of Conventional and Alternative Therapies for HIV Infection and AIDS." *AIDS* 7:561-66.

Andrews, Frank M., Antonia Abbey, and Jill L. Halman. 1991. "Stress from Infertility, Marriage Factors, and Subjective Well-Being of Wives and Husbands." *Journal of Health and Social Behavior* 32:238-53.

Aneshensel, Carol S., Carolyn M. Rutter, and Peter A. Lachenbruch. 1991. "Competing Conceptual and Analytic Models: Social Structure, Stress and Mental Health." *American Sociological Review* 56:166-78.

Angier, Natalie. 1994. "Male Hormone Molds Women, Too, in Mind and Body." *The New York Times,* May 3, pp. C1, C13.

―――. 1995. "Does Testosterone Equal Aggression? Maybe Not." *The New York Times,* June 20, pp. A1, C3.

Anson, Ofra, Arieh Levenson, and Dan Y. Bonneh. 1990. "Gender and Health on the Kibbutz." *Sex Roles* 22:213-35.

Ashley, Jo Ann. 1976. *Hospitals, Paternalism, and the Role of the Nurse.* New York: Teachers College Press.

Atkinson, Paul. 1995. *Medical Talk and Medical Work: The Liturgy of the Clinic.* Thousand Oaks, CA: Sage.

Auerbach, Judith D. and Anne E. Figert. 1995. "Women's Health Research: Public Policy and Sociology." *Journal of Health and Social Behavior* (Extra issue):115-31.

Avis, Nancy E. and Sonja M. McKinlay. 1991. "A Longitudinal Analysis of Women's Attitudes Towards Menopause: Results from the Massachusetts Women's Health Study." *Maturitas* 13:65-79.

―――. 1995. "The Massachusetts Women's Health Study: An Epidemiological Investigation of the Menopause." *Journal of the American Medical Women's Association* 50:45-49, 63.

Bair, Barbara and Susan E. Cayleff, eds. 1993. *Wings of Gauze: Women of Color and the Experience of Health and Illness.* Detroit: Wayne State University Press.

Barefoot Doctor's Manual. 1977. Philadelphia: Running Press.

Barker, Kristen. 1993. "Birthing and Bureaucratic Women: Gender Professionalism and the Construction of Medical Needs, 1920-1935." Ph.D. dissertation, University of Wisconsin, Madison.

Barnett, Elyse Ann. 1988. *"Le Edad Critica:* The Positive Experience of Menopause in a Small Peruvian Town." Pp. 40-54 in *Women and Health: Cross-Cultural Perspectives,* edited by Patricia Whelehan and contributors. Granby, MA: Bergin & Garvey.

Baron, Richard J. 1985. "An Introduction to Medical Phenomenology: I Can't Hear You While I'm Listening." *Annals of Internal Medicine* 103:606-11.

Barr, Kellie E. M., Michael P. Farrell, Grace M. Barnes, and John W. Welte. 1993. "Race, Class, and Gender Differences in Substance Abuse: Evidence of Middle-Class/Underclass Polarization among Black Males." *Social Problems* 40:314-27.

Barroso, Carmen. 1994. "Building a New Specializiation on Women's Health: An International Perspective." Pp. 93-101 in Dan.

Bayer, Ronald. 1994. "Ethical Challenges Posed by Zidovudine Treatment to Reduce Vertical Transmission of HIV." *New England Journal of Medicine* 18:1223-25.

———. 1995. "Women's Rights, Babies' Interests: Ethics, Politics, and Science in the Debate of Newborn HIV Screening." Pp. 293-307 in Minkoff, DeHovitz, and Duerr.

———. 1996. "Rethinking the Testing of Babies and Pregnant Women for HIV Infection." *Journal of Clinical Ethics* 7:85-86.

Bayer, Ronald, N. N. Dubler, and S. Landesman. 1993. "The Dual Epidemics of Tuberculosis and AIDS: Ethical and Policy Issues in Screening and Treatment. *American Journal of Public Health* 83:649-54.

Bayne-Smith, Marcia. 1996. *Race, Gender, and Health.* Thousand Oaks, CA: Sage.

Beckerman, Nancy L., Joan Beder, and Sheldon R. Gelman. 1996. "Mandatory HIV Testing of Newborns: The Debate and a Programmatic Response." *Affilia* 11:462-83.

Bell, Susan E. 1990. "The Medicalization of Menopause." Pp. 43-63 in *The Meaning of Menopause: Historical, Medical, and Clinical Perspectives,* edited by Ruth Formanek. Hillsdale, NJ: Analytic Press.

Berger, J. J., F. Rosner, and P. Farnsworth. 1996. "The Ethics of Mandatory Testing in Newborns." *Journal of Clinical Ethics* 7:77-84.

Bertin, Joan E. 1989. "Women's Health and Women's Rights: Reproductive Hazards in the Workplace." Pp. 289-303 in Ratcliff.

Bevier, Pamela Jean, Mary Ann Chiasson, Richard T. Heffernan, et al. 1995. "Women at a Sexually Transmitted Disease Clinic Who Reported Same-Sex Contact: Their HIV Seroprevalence and Risk Behaviors." *American Journal of Public Health* 85:1366-71.

Bickel, Janet and Phyllis Kopriva. 1993. "A Statistical Perspective on Gender Medicine." *Journal of the American Medical Women's Association* 48:141-44

Biesecker, Barbara Bowles and Lawrence C. Brody. 1997. "Genetic ᶜ Testing for Breast and Ovarian Cancer: A Progress Report." *Jou: Medical Women's Association* 52:22-27.

Bilezikian, John P. and Shonni J. Silverberg. 1992. "Osteoporosis: A Practical Approach to the Perimenopausal Woman." *Journal of Women's Health* 1:21-27.

Bird, Chloe E. and Allen M. Fremont. 1991. "Gender, Time Use, and Health." *Journal of Health and Social Behavior* 32:114-29.

Birke, Linda. 1986. *Women, Feminism and Biology—The Feminist Challenge.* New York: Methuen.

Black, David R., ed. 1991. *Eating Disorders among Athletes.* Reston, VA: American Alliance for Health, Physical Education, Recreation and Dance.

Blackman, Julie. 1989. *Intimate Violence: A Study of Injustice.* New York: Columbia University Press.

Bloor, Michael. 1995. *The Sociology of HIV Transmission.* Thousand Oaks, CA: Sage.

Bond, Lydia S. 1992. "Street Children and AIDS: Is Postponement of Sexual Involvement a Realistic Alternative to the Prevention of Sexually Transmitted Diseases?" *Environment and Urbanization* 4:150-57.

Borchert, Jill and Cheryl A. Rickabaugh. 1995. "When Illness Is Perceived as Controllable: The Effects of Gender and Mode of Transmission on AIDS-Related Stigma." *Sex Roles* 33:657-68.

Bordo, Susan R. 1993. *Unbearable Weight: Feminism, Western Culture, and the Body.* Berkeley: University of California Press.

Borman, A. M., S. Paulous, and F. Clavel. 1996. "Resistance of Human-Immunodeficiency-Virus Type 1 to Protease Inhibitors: Selection of Resistance Mutations in the Presence and Absence of the Drug." *Journal of General Virology* 77(pt. 3):419-26.

Boston Women's Health Book Collective. 1973. *Our Bodies, Ourselves.* New York: Simon & Schuster.

Boyd, Robert L. 1989. "Racial Differences in Childlessness: A Centennial Review." *Sociological Perspectives* 2:183-99.

Bransen, Els. 1992. "Has Menstruation Been Medicalized? Or Will It Never Happen . . . ?" *Sociology of Health and Illness* 14:98-110.

Britton, Carolyn Barley. 1995. "An Argument for Universal HIV Counseling and Voluntary Testing of Women." *Journal of the American Medical Women's Association* 50:85-86.

Brown, Phil. 1995. "Naming and Framing: The Social Construction of Diagnosis and Illness." *Journal of Health and Social Behavior* (Extra issue):34-52.

Browne, J. and V. Minichiello. 1996. "Condoms: Dilemmas of Caring and Autonomy in Heterosexual Safe Sex Practices." *Venereology: Interdisciplinary International Journal of Sexual Health* 9:24-33.

Brumberg, Joan Jacobs. 1988. *Fasting Girls: The Emergence of Anorexia Nervosa as a Modern Disease.* Cambridge, MA: Harvard University Press.

Bryson, Y. J., S. Pang, L. S. Wei, et al. 1995. "Clearance of HIV Infection in a Perinatally Infected Infant." *New England Journal of Medicine* 332:833-38.

Buckley, Thomas and Alma Gottleib. 1988. "A Critical Appraisal of Theories of Menstrual Symbolism." Pp. 3-50 in *Blood Magic: The Anthropology of Menstruation,* edited by Thomas Buckley and Alma Gottleib. Berkeley: University of California Press.

Bullough, Vern and Martha Voght. 1973. "Women, Menstruation and Nineteenth-Century Medicine." *Bulletin of the History of Medicine* 47:66-82.

Burckes-Miller, Mardie E. and David R. Black. 1991. "College Athletes and Eating Disorders: A Theoretical Context." Pp. 11-26 in Black.

Burke, B. Meridith. 1992. "Genetic Counselor Attitudes Towards Fetal Sex Identification and Selective Abortion." *Social Science and Medicine* 34:1263-69.

Bush, Trudy L. 1992. "Feminine Forever Revisited: Menopausal Hormone Therapy in the 1990s." *Journal of Women's Health* 1:1-4.

Butler, Judith. 1993. *Bodies That Matter: On the Discursive Limits of "Sex."* New York: Routledge.

Butter, Irene H., Eugenia S. Carpenter, Bonnie J. Kay, and Ruth S. Simmons. 1987. "Gender Hierarchies in the Health Labor Force." *International Journal of Health Services* 17:133-49.

Butterfield, Fox. 1994. "Teen-Age Homicide Rate Has Soared." *The New York Times,* October 14, p. A22.

Calderone, Karen L. 1990. "The Influence of Gender on the Frequency of Pain and Sedative Medication Administered to Postoperative Patients." *Sex Roles* 23:713-25.

Callahan, Joan C., ed. 1993. *Menopause: A Midlife Passage.* Bloomington: Indiana University Press.

Callan, Victor J., Belinda Kloske, Yoshihisa Kashima, and John F. Hennessey. 1988. "Toward Understanding Women's Decisions to Continue or to Stop *In Vitro* Fertilization: The Role of Social, Psychological, and Background Factors." *Journal of In Vitro Fertilization and Embryo Transfer* 5:363-69.

Calnan, Michael. 1986. "Maintaining Health and Preventing Illness: A Comparison of the Perceptions of Women from Different Social Classes." *Health Promotion* 1:167-77.

Campbell, Carole A. 1990. "Women and AIDS." *Social Science and Medicine* 30:407-15.

———. 1991. "Prostitution, AIDS and Preventive Health Behavior." *Social Science and Medicine* 32:1367-78.

———. 1995. "Male Gender Roles and Sexuality: Implications for Women's AIDS Risk and Prevention." *Social Science and Medicine* 41:197-210.

Candib, Lucy M. 1987. "What Doctors Tell about Themselves to Patients: Implications for Intimacy and Reciprocity in the Relationship." *Family Medicine* 19:23-30.

———. 1988. "Ways of Knowing in Family Medicine: Contributions from a Feminist Perspective." *Family Medicine* 20:133-36.

———. 1995. *Medicine and the Family: A Feminist Perspective.* New York: Basic Books.

Candy, Dana. 1996. "Seeking Assurance from a $40 Kit." *The New York Times,* November 21, pp. D1, D8.

Canetto, Silvia Sara. 1992. "Gender and Suicide in the Elderly." *Suicide and Life Threatening Behavior* 22:80-97.

Chavkin, Wendy, ed. 1994. *Double Exposure: Women's Health Hazards on the Job and at Home.* New York: Monthly Review Press.

Chidambaram, S. Muthu. 1993. "Sex Stereotypes in Women Doctors' Contribution to Medicine in India." Pp. 13-26 in Riska and Wegar.

Chilman, Catherine S. 1989. "Some Major Issues Regarding Adolescent Sexuality and Childbearing in the United States." *Journal of Social Work and Human Sexuality* 8:3-25.

Chodorow, Nancy. 1978. *The Reproduction of Mothering.* Berkeley: University of California Press.

Chrisler, Joan C. and Karen B. Levy. 1990. "The Media Construct a Menstrual Monster: A Content Analysis of PMS Articles in the Popular Press." *Women and Health* 16:69-71.

Chu, Susan Y., J. W. Buehler, P. L. Fleming, and R. L. Berkelman. 1990. "Epidemiology of Reported Cases of AIDS in Lesbians, United States, 1980-89." *American Journal of Public Health* 80:1380-81.

Chu, Susan Y., D. L. Hanson, J. L. Jones, et al. 1996. "Pregnancy Rates Among Women Infected with Human Immunodeficiency Virus." *Obstetrics and Gynecology* 87:195-98.

Chu, Susan Y., T. A. Peterman, L. S. Doll, et al. 1992. "AIDS in Bisexual Men in the United States: Epidemiology and Transmission to Women." *American Journal of Public Health* 82:220-24.

Chu, Susan Y. and Pascale M. Wortley. 1995. "Epidemiology of HIV/AIDS in Women." Pp. 1-12 in Minkoff, DeHovitz, and Duerr.

Cohen, J. 1996. "AIDS Research—Results on New AIDS Drugs Bring Cautious Optimism." *Science* 271 (February 9):755-56.

Cohen, Susan M., Ellen O. Mitchell, Virginia Oleson, et al. 1994. "From Female Disease to Women's Health: New Educational Paradigms." Pp. 50-55 in Dan.

Coleman, Lerita M., Toni C. Antonucci, Pamela K. Adelmann, and Susan E. Chrohan. 1987. "Social Roles in the Lives of Middle-Aged and Older Black Women." *Journal of Marriage and the Family* 49:761-71.

Coleman, Linda and Cindy Dickinson. 1984. "The Risks of Healing: The Hazards of the Nursing Profession." Pp. 37-56 in Chavkin.

Collier, A. C., R. W. Coombs, D. A. Schoenfeld, and R. L. Bassett. 1996. "Treatment of Human-Immunodeficiency-Virus Infection with Saquinavir, Zidovudine, and Zalcitabine: AIDS Clinical Trials Group." *New England Journal of Medicine* 334:1011-17.

Connell, R. W. 1995. *Masculinities.* Berkeley: University of California Press.

Connell, R. W., M. D. Davis, and G. W. Dowsett. 1993. "A Bastard of a Life: Homosexual Desire and Practice among Men in Working-Class Milieux." *Australia and New Zealand Journal of Sociology* 29:112-35.

Connell, R. W. and Susan Kippax. 1990. "Sexuality in the AIDS Crisis: Patterns of Sexual Practice and Pleasure in a Sample of Australian Gay and Bisexual Men." *Journal of Sex Research* 27:167-98.

Connor, E. M., R. S. Sperling, R. Gelber, et al. 1994. "Reduction of Maternal-Infant Transmission of Human Immunodeficiency Virus Type I with Zidovudine Treatment." *New England Journal of Medicine* 331:1173-80.

Conrad, Peter and Joseph W. Schneider. 1992. *Deviance and Medicalization: From Badness to Sickness.* Expanded ed. Philadelphia: Temple University Press.

Coombs, Robert H., Morris J. Paulson, and Mark A. Richardson. 1991. "Peer vs. Parental Influence in Substance Use among Hispanic and Anglo Children and Adolescents." *Journal of Youth and Adolescence* 20:73-88.

Cooper, Elizabeth B. 1995. "Historical and Analytical Overview of Policy Issues Affecting Women Living with AIDS: A Blueprint for Learning from Our Past." *Bulletin of the New York Academy of Medicine* 72(Summer Supp. 1):283-99.

Corea, Gena. 1992. *The Invisible Epidemic: The Story of Women and Aids.* New York: HarperPerennial.

Crossette, Barbara. 1995. "Female Genital Mutilation by Immigrants Is Becoming Cause for Concern in the U.S." *The New York Times,* December 10, Sunday News Section, p. 18.

Crowe, Christine. 1985. " 'Women Want It': *In Vitro* Fertilization and Women's Motivations for Participation." *Women's Studies International Forum* 8:57-62.

Crystal, Stephen and Marguerite Jackson. 1992. "Health Care and the Social Construction of AIDS: The Impact of Disease Definitions." Pp. 163-80 in Huber and Schneider.

Dan, Alice J., ed. 1994. *Reframing Women's Health: Multidisciplinary Research and Practice.* Thousand Oaks, CA: Sage.

Danner, S. W., A. Carr, J. M. Leonard, et al. 1995. "A Short-Term Study of the Safety, Pharmacokinetics, and Efficacy of Ritonavir, an Inhibitor of HIV-1 Protease." *New England Journal of Medicine* 333:1528-33.

Darrow, Sherri L., Marcia Russell, M. Lynne Cooper, et al. 1992. "Sociodemographic Correlates of Alcohol Consumption among African-American and White Women." *Women and Health* 18:35-51.

Daum, Meghan. 1996. "Safe-Sex Lies." *The New York Times Magazine,* January 21, pp. 32-33.

Davis, Kathy. 1988. *Power Under the Microscope.* Dordrecht: Foris.

———. 1995. *Reshaping the Female Body: The Dilemma of Cosmetic Surgery.* New York and London: Routledge.

Dean, Michael, Mary Carrington, Cheryl Winkler, et al. 1996. "Genetic Restriction of HIV-1 Infection and Progression to AIDS by a Deletion Allele of the *CKR5* Structural Gene." *Science* 273(September 27):1856-62.

Delaney, Janice, Mary Jane Lupton, and Emily Toth. 1977. *The Curse: A Cultural History of Menstruation.* New York: New American Library.

Delany, Samuel R. 1991. "Straight Talk/Street Talk." *Differences: A Journal of Feminist Cultural Studies* 3(Summer):21-38.

de Villiers, E. M., C. Dahl, G. Engholm, et al. 1991. "Case Control Study of Risk Factors for Cervical Neoplasia in Denmark. I: Role of the 'Male Factor' in Women with One Lifetime Sexual Partner." *International Journal of Cancer* 48:39-44.

Diamond, Timothy. 1986. "Social Policy and Everyday Life in Nursing Homes: A Critical Ethnography." *Social Science and Medicine* 23:1287-95.

Dickson, Geri L. 1990. "A Feminist Poststructuralist Analysis of the Knowledge of Menopause." *Advances in Nursing Science* 12:15-31.

DiClemente, Ralph J. 1990. "The Emergence of Adolescents as a Risk Group for Human Immunodeficiency Virus Infection." *Journal of Adolescent Research* 5:7-17.

DiClemente, Ralph J. and Gina M. Wingood. 1995. "A Randomized Control Trial of an HIV Sexual Risk-Reduction Intervention for Young African-American Women." *Journal of the American Medical Association* 274:271-76.

Dixon-Mueller, Ruth. 1994. "Abortion Policy and Women's Health in Developing Countries." Pp. 191-210 in Fee and Krieger.

"Doctors Back AIDS Test for Pregnant Women." 1996. *The New York Times,* June 28, p. A20.

Donovan, John E., Richard Jessor, and Frances M. Costa. 1993. "Structure of Health-Enhancing Behavior in Adolescence: A Latent-Variable Approach." *Journal of Health and Social Behavior* 34:346-62.

Douglas, Mary. 1966. *Purity and Danger: An Analysis of the Concepts of Pollution and Taboo.* London: Routledge & Kegan Paul.

Doyal, Lesley. 1995. *What Makes Women Sick: Gender and the Political Economy of Health.* New Brunswick, NJ: Rutgers University Press.

Drachman, Virginia. 1984. *Hospital with a Heart.* Ithaca, New York: Cornell University Press.

Draper, Elaine. 1993. "Fetal Exclusion Policies and Gendered Constructions of Suitable Work." *Social Problems* 40:90-107.

Dugger, Celia W. 1996a. "A Refugee's Body Is Intact but Her Family Is Torn." *The New York Times,* September 11, pp. A1, B6-B7.

———. 1996b. "Genital Ritual Is Unyielding in Africa" *The New York Times,* October 5, Saturday News Section, pp. 1, 6.

———. 1996c. "New Law Bans Genital Cutting in the United States." *The New York Times,* October 12, Saturday News Section, pp. 1, 28.

Duerr, Ann and Gene E. Howe. 1995. "Contraception." Pp. 157-72 in Minkoff, DeHovitz, and Duerr.

Dunlap, David W. 1996a. "From AIDS Conference, Talk of Life, Not Death." *The New York Times,* July 15, p. A7.

———. 1996b. "In Age of AIDS, Love and Hope Can Lead to Risk." *The New York Times,* July 27, p. A7.

———. 1996c. "AIDS Drugs Alter an Industry's Math." *The New York Times,* July 30, pp. D1, D4.

———. 1996d. "Surviving with AIDS: Now What?" *The New York Times,* August 1, pp. C1, C8.

———. 1996e. "For AIDS Doctors, a Needed Tonic." *The New York Times,* September 3, p. D9.

Eckenrode, John and Susan Gore, eds. 1990. *Stress Between Work and Family.* New York: Plenum.

Egan, Timothy. 1996. "Seattle Officials Seeking to Establish a Subsidized Natural Medicine Clinic." *The New York Times*, January 3, p. B1.

Ehrenreich, Barbara and Deirdre English. 1973a. *Witches, Midwives and Nurses: A History of Women Healers.* New York: Feminist Press.

———. 1973b. *Complaints and Disorders: The Sexual Politics of Sickness.* New York: Feminist Press.

El Dareer, Asma. 1982. *Woman, Why Do You Weep? Circumcision and Its Consequences.* London: Zed Books.

Elston, Mary Ann. 1993. "Women Doctors in a Changing Profession: The Case of Britain." Pp. 27-61 in Riska and Wegar.

Erni, John Nguyet. 1994. *Unstable Frontiers: Technomedicine and the Cultural Politics of "Curing" AIDS.* Minneapolis: University of Minnesota Press.

Ettorre, Elizabeth, Timo Klaukka, and Elianne Riska. 1994. "Psychotropic Drugs: Long-Term Use, Dependency and the Gender Factor." *Social Science and Medicine* 12:1667-73.

Ettore, Elizabeth and Elianne Riska. 1995. *Gendered Moods: Psychotropics and Society.* New York: Routledge.

European Collaborative Study. 1991. "Children Born to Women with HIV-1 Infection: Natural History and Risk of Transmission." *Lancet* 337:253-60.

Faden, Ruth R., Gail Geller, and Madison Powers, eds. 1992. *AIDS, Women and the Next Generation: Towards a Morally Acceptable Public Policy for HIV Testing of Pregnant Women and Newborns.* New York: Oxford University Press.

Farberow, Norman L., Dolores Gallagher-Thompson, Michael Gilewski, and Larry Thompson. 1992. "The Role of Social Supports in the Bereavement Process of Surviving Spouses of Suicide and Natural Deaths." *Suicide and Life-Threatening Behavior* 22:107-24.

Farrell, Janice and Kyriakos S. Markides. 1985. "Marriage and Health: A Three-Generation Study of Mexican Americans." *Journal of Marriage and the Family* 47:1029-36.

Fausto-Sterling, Anne. 1985. *Myths of Gender: Biological Theories about Women and Men.* New York: Basic Books.

———. 1993. "The Five Sexes: Why Male and Female Are Not Enough." *The Sciences*, March/April, pp. 20-25.

Featherstone, Mike, Mike Hepworth and Bryan S. Turner, eds. 1991. *The Body: Social Process and Cultural Theory.* London: Sage.

Fee, Elizabeth and Nancy Krieger, eds. 1994a. *Women's Health, Politics, and Power.* Amityville, NY: Baywood.

———. 1994b. "Man-Made Medicine and Women's Health: The Biopolitics of Sex/Gender and Race/Ethnicity." Pp. 11-19 in Fee and Krieger.

Fennelly, Katherine. 1993. "Barriers to Birth Control Use among Hispanic Teenagers: Providers' Perspectives." Pp. 300-11 in Bair and Cayleff.

Fennema, Karen, Daniel L. Meyer, and Natalie Owen. 1990. "Sex of Physician: Patients' Preferences and Stereotypes." *Journal of Family Practice* 30:441-46.

Figert, Anne E. 1995. "The Three Faces of PMS: The Professional, Gendered and Scientific Structuring of a Psychiatric Disorder." *Social Problems* 42:56-73.

Finkelhor, David and Kersti Yllö. 1985. *License to Rape: Sexual Abuse of Wives.* New York: Holt, Rinehart & Winston.

Fisher, Ian. 1996. "To Be Young, Gay, Healthy . . . and Alienated." *The New York Times,* July 14, Sunday News Section, p. 25.

Fisher, Sue. 1986. *In the Patient's Best Interest: Women and the Politics of Medical Decisions.* New Brunswick, NJ: Rutgers University Press.

———. 1994. "Is Care a Remedy? The Case of Nurse Practitioners." Pp. 301-29 in Dan.

———. 1995. *Nursing Wounds: Nurse Practitioners, Doctors, Women Patients, and the Negotiation of Meaning.* New Brunswick, NJ: Rutgers University Press.

Flint, Marcha. 1982. "Male and Female Menopause: A Cultural Put-On." Pp. 363-75 in Voda, Dinnerstein, and O'Donnell.

Flint, Marcha and Ratna Suprapti Samil. 1990. "Cultural and Subcultural Meaning of the Menopause." Pp. 134-48 in *Multidisciplinary Perspectives on Menopause,* edited by Marcha Flint, Fredi Kronenberg, and Wulf Utian. New York: New York Academy of Sciences.

Flitcraft, Anne. 1996. "Synergy: Violence Prevention, Intervention, and Women's Health." *Journal of the American Medical Women's Association* 51:75-76.

Forsyth, Craig J. and Eddie C. Palmer. 1990. "Teenage Pregnancy: Health, Moral and Economic Issues." *International Journal of Sociology of the Family* 20:79-95.

Foster, Johanna. 1996. "Menstrual Time: The Sociocognitive Mapping of 'The Menstrual Cycle.' " *Sociological Forum* 11:523-47.

Foucault, Michel. 1975. *The Birth of the Clinic: An Archeology of Medical Perception.* New York: Vintage.

Fox, Steve. 1991. *Toxic Work: Women Workers at GTE Lenkurt.* Philadelphia: Temple University Press.

Frank, Robert. 1931. "The Hormonal Causes of Premenstrual Tension." *Archives of Neurology and Psychiatry* 26:1053-57.

Franklin, Sara. 1990. "Deconstructing 'Desperateness': The Social Construction of Infertility in Popular Representations of New Reproductive Technologies." Pp. 200-29 in *The New Reproductive Technologies,* edited by M. McNeil, I. Varcoe, and S. Yearley. London: Macmillan.

Franks, Peter and Carolyn M. Clancy. 1993. "Physician Gender Bias in Clinical Decisionmaking: Screening for Cancer in Primary Care." *Medical Care* 31:213-18.

Fraser, Alison M. 1995. "Association of Young Maternal Age with Adverse Reproductive Outcomes." *New England Journal of Medicine* 332:1113-17.

Fraser, Marcy and Diane Jones. 1995. "The Role of Nurses in the HIV Epidemic." Pp. 286-97 in Schneider and Stoller.

Fredericks, Christopher M., John D. Paulson, and Alan H. DeCherney, eds. 1987. *Foundations of In Vitro Fertilization.* Washington, DC: Hemisphere.

Freidson, Eliot. 1970a. *Profession of Medicine.* New York: Dodd, Mead.

———. 1970b. *Professional Dominance: The Social Structure of Medical Care.* New York: Atherton.

———. 1986. *Professional Powers.* Chicago: University of Chicago Press.

———. 1989. *Medical Work in America.* New Haven, CT: Yale University Press.

Fussell, Sam. 1993. "Body Builder Americanus." *Michigan Quarterly Review* 32:577-96.

Gagnon, John. 1992. "Epidemics and Researchers: AIDS and the Practice of Social Studies." Pp. 27-40 in Herdt and Lindenbaum.

Gallagher, Catherine and Thomas Laqueur, eds. 1987. *The Making of the Modern Body.* Berkeley: University of California Press.

Gamble, Vanessa. 1982. "Vanessa Gamble—Tomorrow's Physicians, Tomorrow's Policy-Maker." Pp. 242-61 in *In Her Own Words: Oral Histories of Women Physicians,* edited by Regina Markell Morantz, Cynthia Stodola Pomerlau, and Carol Hensen Fenichel. Westport, CT: Greenwood.

Gamson, Joshua. 1990. "Rubber Wars: Struggles over the Condom in the United States." *Journal of the History of Sexuality* 1:262-82.

Gannon, Linda and Bonnie Ekstrom. 1993. "Attitudes Toward Menopause: The Influence of Sociocultural Paradigms." *Psychology of Women Quarterly* 17:275-88.

Gartner, Rosemary. 1990. "The Victims of Homicide: A Temporal and Cross-National Comparison." *American Sociological Review* 55:92-106.

Gartner, Rosemary, Kathryn Baker, and Fred C. Pampel. 1990. "Gender Stratification and the Gender Gap in Homicide Victimization." *Social Problems* 37:593-612.

Genuis, S. J. and S. K. Genuis. 1996. "Orgasm without Organisms: Science or Propaganda?" *Clinical Pediatrics* 35:10-17.

Gerstel, Naomi and Sally Gallagher. 1994. "Caring for Kith and Kin: Gender, Employment, and the Privatization of Care." *Social Problems* 41:519-39.

Gibbs, Jewelle Taylor, ed. 1988. *Young, Black and Male in America: An Endangered Species.* Dover, MA: Auburn House.

Gitlin, Michael J. and Robert O. Pasnau. 1989. "Psychiatric Syndromes Linked to Reproductive Function in Women: A Review of Current Knowledge." *American Journal of Psychiatry* 146:1413-21.

Glass, Jennifer and Tetsushi Fujimoto. 1994. "Housework, Paid Work, and Depression among Husbands and Wives." *Journal of Health and Social Behavior* 35:179-91.

Glazer, Nona. 1990. "The Home as Workshop: Women as Amateur Nurses and Medical Care Providers." *Gender & Society* 4:479-99.

———. 1991. " 'Between a Rock and Hard Place': Women's Professional Organizations in Nursing and Class, Racial, and Ethnic Inequalities." *Gender & Society* 5:351-72.

Glenn, Evelyn Nakano. 1992. "From Servitude to Service Work: Historical Continuities in the Racial Division of Paid Reproductive Labor." *Signs: Journal of Women in Culture and Society* 18:1-43.

Gold, Ron S., Michael J. Skinner, and Michael W. Ross. 1994. "Unprotected Anal Intercourse in HIV-Infection and Non-HIV-Infected Gay Men." *Journal of Sex Research* 31:59-74.

Goldstein, Nancy. 1995. "Lesbians and the Medical Profession: HIV/AIDS and the Pursuit of Visibility." *Women's Studies* 24:531-52.

Golub, Sharon. 1992. *Periods: From Menarche to Menopause.* Newbury Park, CA: Sage.

Gómez, Cynthia A. 1995. "Lesbians at Risk for HIV: The Unresolved Debate." Pp. 19-31 in *AIDS, Identity, and Community: The HIV Epidemic and Lesbians and Gay Men,* edited by Gregory M. Herek and Beverly Greene. Thousand Oaks, CA: Sage.

Good, Byron J. and Mary-Jo DelVecchio Good. 1993. " 'Learning Medicine': The Constructing of Medical Knowledge at Harvard Medical School." Pp. 81-107 in Lindenbaum and Lock.

Gordon, Linda and Barrie Thorne. 1996. "Women's Bodies and Feminist Subversions." *Contemporary Sociology* 25:322-25.

Gove, Walter R. 1984. "Gender Differences in Mental and Physical Illness: The Effects of Fixed Roles and Nurturant Roles." *Social Science and Medicine* 19:77-91.

Grady, Denise. 1992. "Sex Test of Champions: Olympic Officials Struggle to Define What Should Be Obvious: Just Who Is a Female Athlete?" *Discover* 13(June):78-82.

Graham, Hilary. 1985. "Providers, Negotiators, and Mediators: Women as the Hidden Carers." Pp. 25-52 in *Women, Health, and Healing,* edited by Ellen Lewin and Virginia Oleson. New York: Tavistock.

Green, Jesse. 1996. "Flirting with Suicide." *The New York Times Magazine,* September 15, pp. 39-45, 54-55, 84-85.

Green, Monica. 1989. "Women's Medical Practice and Health Care in Medieval Europe." *Signs: Journal of Women in Culture and Society* 14:434-73.

Greenhalgh, Susan and Jiali Li. 1995. "Engendering Reproductive Policy and Practice in Peasant China: For a Feminist Demography of Reproduction." *Signs: Journal of Women in Culture and Society* 20:601-41.

Greer, Germaine. 1991. *The Change: Women, Aging and the Menopause.* New York: Fawcett Columbine.

Gregersen, Edgar. 1983. *Sexual Practices: The Story of Human Sexuality.* New York: Franklin Watts.

Greil, Arthur L. 1991. *Not Yet Pregnant: Infertile Couples in Contemporary America.* New Brunswick, NJ: Rutgers University Press.

Gross, Jane. 1993. "Second Wave of AIDS Feared by Officials in San Francisco." *The New York Times,* December 11, Sunday News Section, pp. 1, 10.

Guinan, Mary E. 1988. "PMS or Perifollicular Phase Euphoria?" *Journal of the American Medical Women's Association* 43:91-92.

———. 1995. "Artifical Insemination by Donor." *Journal of the American Medical Association* 273:890-91.

Gullette, Margaret Morganroth. 1993. "All Together Now: The New Sexual Politics of Midlife Bodies." *Michigan Quarterly Review* 32:669-95.

Haas, Ann Pollinger. 1994. "Lesbian Health Issues: An Overview." Pp. 339-356 in Dan.

Hall, Judith A., A. M. Epstein, M. L. DeCiantis, and B. J. McNeil. 1993. "Physicians' Liking for Their Patients: More Evidence for the Role of Affect in Medical Care." *Health Psychology* 12:140-46.

Hall, Judith A., Julie T. Irish, Debra L. Roter, et al. 1994. "Gender in Medical Encounters: An Analysis of Physician and Patient Communication in a Primary Care Setting." *Health Psychology* 13:382-92.

Hall, Judith A. and Debra L. Roter. 1995. "Patient Gender and Communication with Physicians: Results of a Community-Based Study." *Women's Health: Research on Gender, Behavior, and Policy* 1:77-95.

Hammonds, Evelynn. 1992. "Missing Persons: African American Women, AIDS and the History of Disease." *Radical America* 24:7-23.

Haraway, Donna. 1981. "In the Beginning Was the Word: The Genesis of Biological Theory." *Signs: Journal of Women in Culture and Society* 6:469-81.

———. 1988. "Situated Knowledges: The Science Question in Feminism and the Privilege of Partial Perspective." *Feminist Studies* 14:575-99.

———. 1989. "The Biopolitics of Postmodern Bodies: Determinations of Self in Immune System Discourse." *Differences: A Journal of Feminist Cultural Studies* 1(Winter):1-43.

Harding, Sandra. 1986. *The Science Question in Feminism.* Ithaca, NY: Cornell University Press.

———. 1991. *Whose Science? Whose Knowledge? Thinking from Women's Lives.* Ithaca, NY: Cornell University Press.

Harlow, Caroline Wolf. 1991. *Female Victims of Violent Crime.* Washington, DC: U.S. Department of Justice, Bureau of Justice Statistics.

Harrison, Michelle. 1983. *A Woman in Residence.* New York: Penguin.

———. 1985. *Self-Help for Premenstrual Syndrome.* New York: Random House.

———. 1994. "Women's Health: New Models of Care and a New Academic Discipline." Pp. 79-90 in Dan.

Hatch, Maureen. 1984. "Mother, Father, Worker: Men and Women and the Reproductive Risks of Work." Pp. 161-79 in Chavkin.

Haug, Marie and Bebe Lavin. 1983. *Consumerism in Medicine: Challenging Physician Authority.* Beverly Hills, CA: Sage.

Healy, Bernadine. 1991. "The Yentl Syndrome." *New England Journal of Medicine* 325:274-76.

Helgeson, Vickie. 1995. "Masculinity, Men's Roles, and Coronary Heart Disease." Pp. 68-104 in Sabo and Gordon.

Hendel, R. C. and M. A. Mendelson. 1995. "Myocardial Infarction in Women." *Cardiology* 86:272-85.

Herdt, Gilbert and Shirley Lindenbaum, eds. 1992. *The Time of AIDS: Social Analysis, Theory, and Method.* Newbury Park, CA: Sage.

Herzog, David B., Isabel Bradburn, and Kerry Newman. 1990. "Sexuality in Males with Eating Disorders." Pp. 40-53 in Andersen.

Herzog, David B., Kerry L. Newman, C. J. Yeh, and Meredith Warshaw. 1992. "Body Image Satisfaction in Homosexual and Heterosexual Women." *International Journal of Eating Disorders* 11:391-96.

Herzog, David B., Dennis K. Norman, Christopher Gordon, and Maura Pepose. 1984. "Sexual Conflict and Eating Disorders in 27 Males." *American Journal of Psychiatry* 141:989-90.

Hesse-Biber, Sharlene J. 1989. "Eating Patterns and Disorders in a College Population: Are College Women's Eating Problems a New Phenomenon?" *Sex Roles* 20:71-89.

Hilts, Philip J. 1995. "Health Maintenance Organizations Turn to Spiritual Healing." *The New York Times*, December 27, p. C10.

Hine, Darlene Clark. 1985. "Co-Laborers in the Work of the Lord: Nineteenth-Century Black Women Physicians." Pp. 107-120 in *"Send Us a Lady Physician": Women Doctors in America, 1835-1920*, edited by Ruth J. Abram. New York: Norton.

———. 1989. *Black Women in White: Racial Conflict and Cooperation in the Nursing Profession, 1890-1950*. New York: Routledge.

Hoffmann, Joan C. 1982. "Biorhythms in Human Reproduction: The Not-So-Steady States." *Signs: Journal of Women in Culture and Society* 7:829-44.

Hogan, Dennis P. and Evelyn M. Kitagawa. 1985. "The Impact of Social Status, Family Structure, and Neighborhood on the Fertility of Black Adolescents." *American Journal of Sociology* 90:825-55.

Hollibaugh, Amber. 1995. "Lesbian Denial and Lesbian Leadership in the AIDS Epidemic: Bravery and Fear in the Construction of Lesbian Geography of Risk." Pp. 219-30 in Schneider and Stoller.

Horton, Claire F. 1984. "Women Have Headaches, Men Have Backaches: Patterns of Illness in an Appalachian Community." *Social Science and Medicine* 19:647-54.

Horsman, Janet M. and Paschal Sheeran. 1995. "Health Care Workers and HIV/AIDS: A Critical Review of the Literature." *Social Science and Medicine* 41:1535-67.

Horwitz, Allan V., Helene Raskin White, and Sandra Howell-White. 1996. "The Use of Multiple Outcomes in Stress Research: A Case Study of Gender Differences in Responses to Marital Dissolution." *Journal of Health and Social Behavior* 37:278-91.

Hsia, Judith. 1993. "Gender Differences in Diagnosis and Management of Coronary Heart Disease." *Journal of Women's Health* 2:349-52.

Hubbard, Ruth. 1990. *The Politics of Women's Biology*. New Brunswick, NJ: Rutgers University Press.

Huber, Joan and Beth E. Schneider, eds. 1992. *The Social Context of AIDS*. Newbury Park, CA: Sage.

Hutchinson, Margaret and Maureen Shannon. 1993. "Reproductive Health and Counseling." Pp. 47-65 in Kurth.

Idler, Ellen L. and Stanislav V. Kasl. 1992. "Religion, Disability, Depression, and the Timing of Death." *American Journal of Sociology* 97:1052-79.

Irigaray, Luce. [1977] 1985. *This Sex Which Is Not One*. Translated by Catherine Porter with Carolyn Burke. Ithaca, NY: Cornell University Press.

Jaccard, James J., Tracey E. Wilson, and Carmen M. Radecki. 1995. "Psychological Issues in the Treatment of HIV-Infected Women." Pp. 87-105 in Minkoff, DeHovitz, and Duerr.

Jason, J., B. L. Evatt, and Hemophilia-AIDS Collaborative Study Group. 1990. "Pregnancies in Human Immunodeficiency Virus-Infected Sex Partners of Hemophilic Men." *American Journal of Diseases of Children* 144:485-90.

Johnson, Karen and Eileen Hoffman. 1994. "Women's Health and Curriculum Transformation: The Role of Medical Specialization." Pp. 27-39 in Dan.

Johnson, Richard E. and Anastasios C. Marcos. 1988. "Correlates of Adolescent Drug Use by Gender and Geographic Location." *American Journal of Drug and Alcohol Abuse* 14:51-63.

Johnson, Valerie. 1988. "Adolescent Alcohol and Marijuana Use: A Longitudinal Assessment of a Social Learning Perspective." *American Journal of Drug and Alcohol Abuse* 14:419-39.

Jonas, Harry S. and Sylvia I. Etzel. 1988. "Undergraduate Medical Education." *Journal of the American Medical Association* 260:1063-71.

Jonas, Helen A. and Teri A. Manolio. 1996. "Hormone Replacement and Cardiovascular Disease in Older Women." *Journal of Women's Health* 5:351-61.

Jones, Elise and Jacqueline Darroch Forrest. 1985. "Teenage Pregnancy in Developed Countries: Determinants and Policy Implications." *Family Planning Perspectives* 17:53-63.

Jones, Wanda, Dixie E. Snider, and Rueben C. Warren. 1996. "Deciphering the Data: Race, Ethnicity, and Gender as Critical Variables." *Journal of the American Medical Women's Association* 51:137-38.

Jordanova, Ludmilla. 1989. *Sexual Visions: Images of Gender in Science and Medicine between the Eighteenth and Twentieth Centuries.* Madison: University of Wisconsin Press.

Joseph, Stephen C. 1992. *Dragon within the Gates: The Once and Future AIDS Epidemic.* New York: Carroll & Graf.

Kauppinen-Toropainen, Kaisa and Johanna Lammi. 1993. "Men in Female-Dominated Occupations: A Cross-Cultural Comparison." Pp. 91-112 in *Doing "Women's Work": Men in Nontraditional Occupations,* edited by Christine Williams. Newbury Park, CA: Sage.

Kane, Stephanie and Theresa Mason. 1992. " 'IV Drug Users' and 'Sex Partners': The Limits of Epidemiological Categories and the Ethnography of Risk." Pp. 199-222 in Herdt and Lindenbaum.

Kassler, W. J., P. Blanc, and R. Greenblatt. 1991. "The Use of Medicinal Herbs by Human Immunodeficiency Virus-Infected Patients." *Archives of Internal Medicine* 151:2281-88.

Kearney-Cooke, Ann and Paule Steichen-Asch. 1990. "Men, Body Image, and Eating Disorders." Pp. 54-74 in Andersen.

Keller, Evelyn Fox. 1985. *Reflections on Gender and Science.* New Haven, CT: Yale University Press.

Kelly, J. A., J. S. St. Lawrence, Y. E. Diaz, et al. 1991. "HIV Risk Behavior Reduction Following Intervention with Key Opinion Leaders of a Population: An

Experimental Community-Level Analysis." *American Journal of Public Health* 81:168-71.

Kelly, Jeffrey A. 1995a. "Advances in HIV/AIDS Education and Prevention." *Family Relations* 44:345-52.

———. 1995b. *Changing HIV Risk Behavior: Practical Strategies*. New York: Guilford.

Kelly, J., J. Lawrence, H. Hood, and T. Brasfield. 1989. "HIV Risk Reduction Following Intervention with Key Opinion Leaders of Population: An Experimental Analysis." *American Journal of Public Health* 81:168-71.

Kelly, Patricia J. 1995. "Starting a Clinic for Women with HIV Disease." Pp. 279-91 in Minkoff, DeHovitz, and Duerr.

Kemp, Alice Abel and Pamela Jenkins. 1992. "Gender and Technological Hazards: Women at Risk in Hospital Settings." *Industrial Crisis Quarterly* 6:137-52.

Kemper, Theodore D. 1990. *Social Structure and Testosterone: Explorations of the Socio-Bio-Social Chain*. New Brunswick, NJ: Rutgers University Press.

Kennedy, Meaghan B., Margaret I. Scarlett, Ann C. Duerr, and Susan Y. Chu. 1995. "Assessing HIV Risk Among Women Who Have Sex with Women: Scientific and Communication Issues." *Journal of the American Medical Women's Association* 50:103-07.

Kessler, R. C., C. Foster, F. E. Norlock, et al. 1993. "Unconventional Medicine in the United States: Prevalence, Costs, and Patterns of Use." *New England Journal of Medicine* 328:246-52.

Kimmel, Michael and Martin P. Levine. 1991. "A Hidden Factor in AIDS: 'Real' Men's Hypersexuality." *Los Angeles Times*, June 3, p. B5.

King, Donna. 1990. "Prostitutes as Pariah in the Age of AIDS: A Content Analysis of Coverage of Women Prostitutes in *The New York Times* and *The Washington Post*, September 1985-April 1988." *Women and Health* 16:135-76.

Kliewer, Erich V. and Ken R. Smith. 1995. "Breast Cancer Mortality among Immigrants in Australia and Canada." *Journal of the National Cancer Institute* 87:1154-61.

Klinge, Ineke. 1996. "Female Bodies and Brittle Bones: An Analysis of Intervention Practices for Osteoporosis." *European Journal of Women's Studies* 3:269-83.

Knight, Chris. 1991. *Blood Relations: Menstruation and the Origins of Culture*. New Haven, CT: Yale University Press.

Koch, Lene. 1990. "IVF—An Irrational Choice?" *Issues in Reproductive and Genetic Engineering* 3:235-42.

Koeske, Randi Daimon. 1983. "Lifting the Curse of Menstruation: Toward a Feminist Perspective on the Menstrual Cycle." *Women and Health* 8(2-3):1-15.

Kolata, Gina. 1991. "Hit Hard by AIDS Virus, Hemophiliacs Angrily Speak Out." *The New York Times*, December 25, p. A7.

———. 1996. "On Fringes of Health Care, Untested Therapies Thrive." *The New York Times*, June 17, pp. A1, B6.

Koos, E. L. 1954. *The Health of Regionville*. New York: Columbia University Press.

Korvick, Joyce A., Pamela Stratton, Cathie Spino, et al. 1996. "Women's Participation in AIDS Clinical Trials Group (ACTG) Trials in the USA: Enough or Still Too Few?" *Journal of Women's Health* 5:129-36.

Kramer, Larry. 1996. "A Good News/Bad News AIDS Joke." *The New York Times Magazine*, July 14, pp. 26-29.

Kranczer, Stanley. 1995. "U.S. Longevity Unchanged." *Statistical Bulletin* 76(3):12-20.

Kreuter, Matthew W., Victor J. Strecher, Russell Harris et al. 1995. "Are Patients of Women Physicians Screened More Aggressively? A Prospective Study of Physician Gender and Screening." *Journal of General Internal Medicine* 10:119-25.

Krieger, Nancy. 1996. "Inequality, Diversity, and Health: Thoughts on 'Race/Ethnicity' and 'Gender.' " *Journal of the American Medical Women's Association* 51:133-36.

Kristiansen, Connie M. 1989. "Gender Differences in the Meaning of Health." *Social Behavior* 4:185-88.

Kurth, Ann, ed. 1993. *Until the Cure: Caring for Women with HIV*. New Haven, CT: Yale University Press.

Kurz, Demie. 1987. "Emergency Department Response to Battered Women: A Case of Resistance." *Social Problems* 34:501-13.

Lai, Gina. 1995. "Work and Family Roles and Psychological Well-Being in Urban China." *Journal of Health and Social Behavior* 36:11-37.

Laqueur, Thomas. 1990. *Making Sex: Body and Gender from the Greeks to Freud.* Cambridge, MA: Harvard University Press.

Larson, Magali Sarfati. 1977. *The Rise of Professionalism*. Berkeley: University of California Press.

Lasker, Judith N. and Shirley Borg. 1995. *In Search of Parenthood: Coping with Infertility and High-Tech Conception*. Philadelphia: Temple University Press.

Latour, Bruno. 1987. *Science in Action*. Cambridge, MA: Harvard University Press.

Laumann, Edward O., John H. Gagnon, and Stuart Michaels. 1993. "Monitoring AIDS and Other Rare Population Events: A Network Approach." *Journal of Health and Social Behavior* 34:7-22.

Laws, Sophie. 1983. "The Sexual Politics of Premenstrual Tension." *Women's Studies International Forum* 6:19-31.

———. 1990. *Issues of Blood: The Politics of Menstruation*. London: Macmillan.

Laws, Sophie, Valerie Hey, and Andrea Egan. 1985. *Seeing Red: The Politics of Premenstrual Tension*. London: Hutchinson.

Lazarus, Ellen. 1988a. "Poor Women, Poor Outcomes: Social Class and Reproductive Health." Pp. 39-54 in *Childbirth in America*, edited by Karen L. Michaelson. South Hadley, MA: Bergin & Garvey.

———. 1988b. "Theoretical Considerations for the Study of the Doctor-Patient Relationship: Implications of a Perinatal Study." *Medical Anthropology Quarterly* 2:34-58.

———. 1990. "Falling Through the Cracks: Contradictions and Barriers to Care in a Perinatal Clinic." *Medical Anthropology* 12:269-87.

————. 1994. "What Do Women Want? Issues of Choice, Control, and Class in Pregnancy and Childbirth." *Medical Anthropology Quarterly* 8:25-46.

Lear, Dana. 1995. "Sexual Communication in the Age of AIDS: The Construction of Risk and Trust among Young Adults." *Social Science and Medicine* 41:1311-23.

Lennane, K. Jean and R. John Lennane. 1973. "Alleged Psychogenic Disorders in Women—A Possible Manifestation of Sexual Prejudice." *New England Journal of Medicine* 288:288-92.

Lennon, Mary Clare. 1994. "Women, Work, and Well-Being: The Importance of Work Conditions." *Journal of Health and Social Behavior* 35:235-47.

Lennon, Mary Clare and Sara Rosenfeld. 1992. "Women and Mental Health: The Interaction of Job and Family Conditions." *Journal of Health and Social Behavior* 33:31-27.

Leslie, Charles, ed. 1976. *Asian Medical Systems.* Berkeley: University of California Press.

Levesque-Lopman, Louise. 1988. *Claiming Reality: Phenomenology and Women's Experience.* Totowa, NJ: Rowman & Littlefield.

Levine, Carol. 1993. "Ethical Issues." Pp. 112-24 in Kurth.

Levine, Carol and Nancy Neveloff Dubler. 1990. "Uncertain Risks and Bitter Realities: The Reproductive Choices of HIV-Infected Women." *Millbank Quarterly* 68:321-51.

Levine, Martin P. 1992. "The Implications of Constructionist Theory for Social Research on the AIDS Epidemic among Gay Men." Pp. 185-98 in Herdt and Lindenbaum.

Levine, Martin P. and Karolynn Siegel. 1992. "Unprotected Sex: Understanding Gay Men's Participation." Pp. 47-71 in Huber and Schneider.

Lewin, Ellen and Virginia Olesen. 1985. *Women, Health, and Healing.* New York: Tavistock.

Lewis, Diane K. 1995. "African-American Women at Risk: Notes on the Sociocultural Context of HIV Infection." Pp. 57-73 in Schneider and Stoller.

Lewis, Jane. 1993. "Feminism, the Menopause and Hormone Replacement Therapy." *Feminist Review* 43:38-56.

Lieberman, Ellice, Kenneth J. Ryan, Richard R. Monson, and Stephen C. Schoenbaum. 1987. "Risk Factors Accounting for Racial Differences in the Rate of Premature Birth." *New England Journal of Medicine* 317:743-48.

Lightfoot-Klein, Hanny. 1989. *Prisoners of Ritual: An Odyssey into Female Circumcision in Africa.* New York: Harrington Park Press.

Lillard, Lee A. and Linda J. Waite. 1995. " 'Til Death Do Us Part: Marital Disruption and Mortality." *American Journal of Sociology* 100:1131-56.

Lindenbaum, Shirley and Margaret Lock, eds. 1993. *Knowledge, Power and Practice: The Anthropology of Medicine and Everyday Life.* Berkeley: University of California Press.

Link, Bruce G. and Jo Phelan. 1995. "Social Conditions as Fundamental Causes of Disease." *Journal of Health and Social Behavior* (Extra issue):80-94.

Liu, Rong, William A. Paxton, Sunny Choe, et al. 1996. "Homozygous Defect in HIV-1 Coreceptor Accounts for Resistance of Some Multiply-Exposed Individuals to HIV-1 Infection." *Cell* 86:367-77.

Lock, Margaret. 1993. *Encounters with Aging: Mythologies of Menopause in Japan and North America.* Berkeley: University of California Press.

Longino, Charles F., Jr. 1988. "A Population Profile of Very Old Men and Women in the United States." *Sociological Quarterly* 29:559-64.

Longino, Helen E. 1990. *Science as Social Knowledge: Values and Objectivity in Scientific Inquiry.* Princeton, NJ: Princeton University Press.

Lorber, Judith. 1975a. "Women and Medical Sociology: Invisible Professionals and Ubiquitous Patients." Pp. 75-105 in *Another Voice: Feminist Perspectives on Social Life and Social Science,* edited by Marcia Millman and Rosabeth Moss Kanter. Garden City, NY: Doubleday/Anchor.

———. 1975b. "Good Patients and Problem Patients: Conformity and Deviance in a General Hospital." *Journal of Health and Social Behavior* 16:213-25.

———. 1984. *Women Physicians: Careers, Status, and Power.* New York and London. Tavistock.

———. 1985. "More Women Physicians: Will It Mean More Humane Health Care?" *Social Policy* 16(Summer):50-54.

———. 1987. "*In Vitro* Fertilization and Gender Politics." *Women & Health* 13:117-33.

———. 1989. "Choice, Gift, or Patriarchal Bargain? Women's Consent to *In Vitro* Fertilization in Male Infertility." *Hypatia* 4:23-36.

———. 1993a. "Why Women Physicians Will Never Be True Equals in the American Medical Profession." Pp. 62-97 in Riska and Wegar.

———1993b. "Believing Is Seeing: Biology as Ideology." *Gender & Society* 7:568-81.

———. 1994. *Paradoxes of Gender.* New Haven, CT: Yale University Press.

Lorber, Judith and Lakshmi Bandlamudi. 1993. "Dynamics of Marital Bargaining in Male Infertility." *Gender & Society* 7:32-49.

Lorber, Judith and Dorothy Greenfeld. 1990. "Couples' Experiences with *In Vitro* Fertilization: A Phenomenological Approach. Pp. 965-71 in *Advances in Assisted Reproductive Technologies,* edited by S. Mashiach et al. New York: Plenum.

Loscosso, Karyn A. and Glenna Spitze. 1990. "Working Conditions, Social Support, and the Well-Being of Female and Male Factory Workers." *Journal of Health and Social Behavior* 31:313-27.

Luker, Kristin. 1996. *Dubious Conceptions: The Politics of Teen Pregnancy.* Cambridge, MA: Harvard University Press.

Lupton, Deborah. 1993. "Risk as Moral Danger: The Social and Political Functions of Risk Discourse in Public Health." *International Journal of Health Services* 23:425-35.

Lupton, Deborah, Sophie McCarthy, and Simon Chapman. 1995. " 'Panic Bodies': Discourses on Risk and HIV Antibody Testing." *Sociology of Health and Illness* 17:89-108.

Lurie, Nicole, Jonathan Slater, Paul McGovern, et al. 1993. "Preventive Care for Women: Does the Sex of the Physician Matter?" *New England Journal of Medicine* 329:478-82.

MacFarqhar, Neil. 1996. "Mutilation of Egyptian Girls: Despite Ban, It Goes On." *The New York Times*, August 8, p. A3.

Maddi, Salvatore R. and Suzanne C. Kobasa. 1984. *The Hardy Executive: Health under Stress.* Homewood, IL: Dow Jones-Irwin.

Madigan, M. Patricia, Regina G. Ziegler, Jacques Benichou, et al. 1995. "Proportion of Breast Cancer Cases in the United States Explained by Well-Established Risk Factors." *Journal of the National Cancer Institute* 87:1681-85.

Mansfield, Alan and Barbara McGinn. 1993. "Pumping Irony: The Muscular and the Feminine." Pp. 49-68 in *Body Matters: Essays on the Sociology of the Body*, edited by Sue Scott and David Morgan. London: Falmer.

Markens, Susan. 1996. "The Problematic of 'Experience': A Political and Cultural Critique of PMS." *Gender & Society* 10:42-58.

Markowitz, M., M. Saag, W. G. Powderly, et al. 1995. "A Preliminary Study of Ritonavir, an Inhibitor of HIV-1 Protease, to Treat HIV-1 Infection." *New England Journal of Medicine* 333:1534-39.

Marsiglio, William. 1988. "Commitment to Social Fatherhood: Predicting Adolescent Males' Intentions to Live with Their Child and Partner." *Journal of Marriage and the Family* 50:427-41.

Martin, Emily. [1987] 1992. *The Woman in the Body: A Cultural Analysis of Reproduction.* Boston: Beacon.

————. 1994. *Flexible Bodies: The Role of Immunity in American Culture from the Days of Polio to the Age of AIDS.* Boston: Beacon.

Martin, Steven C., Robert M. Arnold, and Ruth M. Parker. 1988. "Gender and Medical Socialization." *Journal of Health and Social Behavior* 29:333-43.

Massad, L. Stewart, Mary S. Farhi, Lori E. Ackatz, et al. 1995. "Sexual Behaviors of Heterosexual Women Infected with HIV." *Journal of Women's Health* 4:681-84.

Mastroianni, Anna C., Ruth Faden, and Daniel Federman, eds. 1994. *Women and Health Research: Ethical and Legal Issues of Including Women in Clinical Studies.* Washington, DC: National Academy Press.

Masur, Henry, M. A. Michelis, G. P. Wormser, et al. 1982. "Opportunistic Infection in Previously Healthy Women: Initial Manifestation of a Community-Acquired Cellular Immunodeficiency." *Annals of Internal Medicine* 97:533-38.

Mbizvo, M. T. and M. T. Basset. 1996. "Reproductive Health and AIDS Prevention in Sub-Saharan Africa: The Case for Increased Male Participation." *Health Policy and Planning* 11:84-92.

McClintock, Martha K. 1971. "Menstrual Synchrony and Suppression." *Nature* 229:244-45.

McCrea, Frances B. 1986. "The Politics of Menopause: The 'Discovery' of a Deficiency Disease." Pp. 296-307 in *The Sociology of Health and Illness*, edited by Peter Conrad and Rochelle Kern. New York: St. Martin's.

McGovern, Theresa, Martha Davis, and Mary Beth Caschetta. 1994. "Inclusion of Women in AIDS Clinical Research: A Political and Legal Analysis." *Journal of the American Medical Women's Association* 49:102-04, 109.

McKinlay, John B. 1996. "Some Contributions from the Social System to Gender Inequalities in Heart Disease." *Journal of Health and Social Behavior* 37:1-26.

Mellors, J. W. 1996. "Closing in on Human Immunodeficiency Virus-1." *Nature Medicine* 2(March):274-75.

Melnick, Sandra L., Renslow Sherer, Thomas A. Louis, et al. 1994. "Survival and Disease Progression According to Gender of Patients with HIV Infection." *Journal of the American Medical Association* 272:1915-21.

Melosh, Barbara. 1982. *"The Physician's Hand": Work Culture and Conflict in American Nursing.* Philadelphia: Temple University Press.

Merrick, Janna C. and Robert H. Blank. 1993. *The Politics of Pregnancy: Policy Dilemmas in the Maternal-Fetal Relationship.* New York: Haworth.

Mertz, D., M. A. Sushinsky, and U. Schuklenk. 1996. "Women and AIDS: The Ethics of Exaggerated Harm." *Bioethics* 10:93-113.

Messner, Michael. 1992. *Power at Play: Sports and the Problem of Masculinity.* Boston: Beacon.

Miall, Charlene E. 1986. "The Stigma of Involuntary Childlessness." *Social Problems* 33:268-82.

Minkoff, Howard. 1995. "Pregnancy and HIV Infection." Pp. 173-88 in Minkoff, DeHovitz, and Duerr.

Minkoff, Howard, Jack A. DeHovitz, and Ann Duerr, eds. 1995. *HIV Infection in Women.* New York: Raven Press.

Mishler, Elliot G. 1981. "Viewpoint: Critical Perspectives on the Biomedical Model." Pp. 1-23 in *Social Contexts of Health, Illness, and Patient Care,* edited by Elliot G. Mishler et al. Cambridge, UK: Cambridge University Press.

———. 1984. *The Discourse of Medicine: Dialectics of Medical Interviews.* Norwood, NJ: Ablex.

Moldow, Gloria. 1987. *Women Doctors in Gilded-Age Washington: Race, Gender, and Professionalization.* Urbana and Chicago: University of Illinois Press.

Moneyham, Linda, Brenda Seals, Alice Demi, et al. 1996. "Experiences of Disclosure in Women Infected with HIV." *Health Care for Women International* 17:209-21.

Morantz, Regina M. and Sue Zschoche. 1980. "Professionalism, Feminism, and Gender Roles: A Comparative Study of Nineteenth Century Medical Therapeutics." *Journal of American History* 68:568-88.

Morantz-Sanchez, Regina M. 1985. *Sympathy and Science: Women Physicians in American Medicine.* New York: Oxford University Press.

Morgan, John H. 1983. *Third World Medicine and Social Change.* Lanham, MD: University Press of America.

Muller, Charlotte. 1990. *Health Care and Gender.* New York: Russell Sage.

Muncy, Robyn. 1991. *Creating a Female Dominion in American Reform, 1890-1935.* New York: Oxford University Press.

Nachtigall, Lila E. and Lisa B. Nachtigall. 1995. "Estrogen Issues in Relation to Cardiovascular Disease." *Journal of the American Medical Women's Association* 50:7-10.

Nachtigall, Robert D., Gay Becker, and Mark Wozny. 1992. "The Effects of Gender-Specific Diagnosis on Men's and Women's Responses to Infertility." *Fertility and Sterility* 57:113-21.

Nam, Charles B., Isaac W. Eberstein, and Larry C. Deeb. 1989. "Sudden Infant Death Syndrome as a Socially Determined Cause of Death." *Social Biology* 36:1-8.

Navarro, Mireya. 1991. "Epidemic Changes All at Inner-City Medical Center." *The New York Times*, November 11, pp. A1, B2.

———. 1995. "Women in Puerto Rico Find Marriage No Haven from AIDS." *The New York Times*, January 20, p. A14.

Neigus, Alan, Samuel R. Friedman, Richard Curtis, et al. 1994. "The Relevance of Drug Injectors' Social and Risk Networks for Understanding and Preventing HIV Infection." *Social Science and Medicine* 38:67-78.

Nechas, Eileen and Denise Foley. 1994. *Unequal Treatment: What You Don't Know about How Women are Mistreated by the Medical Community.* New York: Simon & Schuster.

Nicolosi, A., M. Leite, M. Musico, et al. 1994. "The Efficiency of Male-to-Female and Female-to-Male Transmission of the Human Immunodeficiency Virus: A Study of 730 Stable Couples." *Epidemiology* 5:570-75.

Nosek, Margaret A. 1992. "Primary Care Issues for Women with Severe Disabilities." *Journal of Women's Health* 1:245-48.

Nosek, Margaret A., Mary Ellen Young, Diana H. Rintala, et al. 1995. "Barriers to Reproductive Health Maintenance among Women with Physical Disabilities." *Journal of Women's Health* 4:505-18.

Notzer, Netta and S. Brown. 1995. "The Feminization of the Medical Profession in Israel." *Medical Education* 29:377-81.

Novello, Antonia Coello. 1995. "Introduction: Women and AIDS." Pp. xi-xiv in Minkoff, DeHovitz, and Duerr.

Nsiah-Jefferson, Laurie and Elaine J. Hall. 1989. "Reproductive Technology: Perspectives and Implications for Low-Income Women and Women of Color." Pp. 93-117 in Ratcliff.

Nyamathi, Adeline and Rose Vasquez. 1989. "Impact of Poverty, Homelessness, and Drugs on Hispanic Women at Risk for HIV Infection." *Hispanic Journal of Behavioral Sciences* 11:299-314.

O'Hanlan, Katherine A. 1995. "Lesbian Health and Homophobia: Perspectives for the Treating Obstetrician/Gynecologist." *Current Problems in Obstetrics, Gynecology and Fertility* 18:94-133.

Oleckno, William A. and Michael J. Blacconiere. 1990. "Wellness of College Students and Differences by Gender, Race, and Class Standing." *College Student Journal* 24:421-29.

O'Neill, John. 1985. *Five Bodies: The Human Shape of Modern Society.* Ithaca, NY: Cornell University Press.

————. 1989. *The Communicative Body: Studies in Communicative Philosophy, Politics, and Sociology.* Evanston, IL: Northwestern University Press.

Orden, Susan R., Kiang Liu, Karen J. Ruth, David R. Jacobs, Jr., et al. 1995. "Multiple Social Roles and Blood Pressure of Black and White Women: The CARDIA Study." *Journal of Women's Health* 4:281-91.

Osmond, Marie Withers, K. G. Wambach, Diane Harrison, et al. 1993. "The Multiple Jeopardy of Race, Class, and Gender for AIDS Risk among Women." *Gender & Society* 7:99-120.

Ouellette, Suzanne K. 1993. "Inquiries into Hardiness." Pp. 77-100 in *Handbook of Stress: Theoretical and Clinical Aspects*, 2nd ed., edited by L. Goldberger and S. Breznitz. New York: Free Press.

Paauw, D. S., D. H. Spach, and J. I. Wallace. 1993. "HIV Infection in Older Patients: When to Suspect the Unexpected." *Geriatrics* 48:61-64, 69-70.

Padian, Nancy S., L. Marquis, D. P. Francis, et al. 1987. "Male-to-Female Transmission of Human Immunodeficiency Virus." *Journal of the American Medical Association* 258:788-90.

Padian, Nancy S., S. C. Shiboski, and N. P. Jewell. 1991. "Female-to-Male Transmission of Human Immunodeficiency Virus." *Journal of the American Medical Association* 266:1664-67.

Palermo, G. D., J. Cohen, and Z. Rosenwaks. 1996. "Intracytoplasmic Sperm Injection a Powerful Tool to Overcome Fertilization Failure." *Fertility and Sterility* 65:899-908.

Park, Robert L. and Ursula Goodenough. 1996. "Buying Snake Oil with Tax Dollars." *The New York Times*, January 3, p. A15.

Parker, Richard C. 1992. "Sexual Diversity, Cultural Analsysis, and AIDS Education in Brazil." Pp. 225-42 in Herdt and Lindenbaum.

Parlee, Mary Brown. 1973. "The Premenstrual Syndrome." *Psychological Bulletin.* 80:454-65.

————. 1982a. "The Psychology of the Menstrual Cycle: Biological and Psychological Perspectives." Pp. 77-99 in *Behavior and the Menstrual Cycle*, edited by Richard C. Friedman. New York: Marcel Dekker.

————. 1982b. "Changes in Moods and Activation Levels During the Menstrual Cycle in Experimentally Naive Subjects." *Psychology of Women Quarterly* 7:119-31.

————. 1994. "The Social Construction of Premenstrual Syndrome: A Case Study of Scientific Discourse as Cultural Contestation." Pp. 91-107 in *The Good Body: Asceticism in Contemporary Culture*, edited by Mary G. Winkler and Letha B. Cole. New Haven, CT: Yale University Press.

Parsons, Talcott. 1951. *The Social System.* New York: Free Press.

Patton, Cindy. 1994. *Last Served? Gendering the HIV Pandemic.* London: Taylor & Francis.

Perkins, H. Wesley. 1992. "Gender Patterns in Consequences of Collegiate Alcohol Abuse: A 10-Year Study of Trends in an Undergraduate Population." *Journal of Studies on Alcohol* 53:458-62.

Pescosolido, Bernice A. 1992. "Beyond Rational Choice: The Social Dynamics of How People Seek Help." *American Journal of Sociology* 97:1096-138.

Pfeffer, Naomi. 1987. "Artificial Insemination, *In vitro* Fertilization and the Stigma of Infertility." Pp. 81-97 in *Reproductive Technologies: Gender, Motherhood and Medicine*, edited by Michelle Stanworth. Minneapolis: University of Minnesota Press.

Phillips, David P. and Kenneth A. Feldman. 1973. "A Dip in Deaths Before Ceremonial Occasions: Some New Relationships between Social Integration and Mortality." *American Sociological Review* 38:678-96.

Phillips, David P. and Elliot W. King. 1988. "Death Takes a Holiday: Mortality Surrounding Major Social Occasions." *Lancet* 337:728-32.

Phillips, David P., Todd E. Ruth, and Lisa M. Wagner. 1993. "Psychology and Survival." *Lancet* 342:1142-45.

Phillips, David P. and Daniel G. Smith. 1990. "Postponement of Death Until Symbolically Meaningful Occasions." *Journal of the American Medical Association* 263:1947-51.

Pies, Cheri. 1995. "AIDS, Ethics, Reproductive Rights: No Easy Answers." Pp. 322-34 in Schneider and Stoller.

Pivnick, Anitra. 1991. "Reproductive Decisions among HIV-Infected, Drug-Using Women: The Importance of Mother-Child Coresidence." *Medical Anthropology Quarterly* 5:153-69.

Popay, Jennie. 1992. " 'My Health Is All Right, But I'm Just Tired All the Time': Women's Experience of Ill Health." Pp. 99-120 in *Women's Health Matters*, edited by Helen Roberts. New York: Routledge.

Prior, Jerilynn C., Yvette M. Vigna, Martin T. Schechter, and Arthur E. Burgess. 1990. "Spinal Bone Loss and Ovulatory Disturbances." *New England Journal of Medicine* 323:1221-27.

Profet, Margie. 1993. "Menstruation as a Defense Against Pathogens Transported by Sperm." *Quarterly Review of Biology* 68:335-81.

Ptacek, James. 1988. "Why Do Men Batter Their Wives? Pp. 133-57 in *Feminist Perspectives on Wife Abuse*, edited by Kersti Yllö and Michele Bograd. Newbury Park, CA: Sage.

Pugliesi, Karen. 1995. "Work and Well-Being: Gender Differences in the Psychological Consequences of Employment." *Journal of Health and Social Behavior* 36:57-71.

Ratcliff, Kathryn Strother, ed. 1989. *Healing Technology: Feminist Perspectives*. Ann Arbor: University of Michigan Press.

Ray, Lawrence J. 1989. "AIDS as a Moral Metaphor: An Analysis of the Politics of the 'Third Epidemic.' " *European Journal of Sociology* 30:243-73.

Redmond, Marcia A. 1985. "Attitudes of Adolescent Males toward Adolescent Pregnancy and Fatherhood." *Family Relations* 34:337-42.

Reeves, W. C., M. M. Brenes, R. Herrero, et al. 1989. "The Male Factor in the Etiology of Cervical Cancer among Sexually Monogamous Women." *International Journal of Cancer* 44:199-203.

Reid, Elizabeth. 1990. "Young Women and the HIV Epidemic." *Development* 1:16-19.

Reiser, Stanley Joel. 1978. *Medicine and the Reign of Technology*. Cambridge, UK: Cambridge University Press.

Renteln, Alison Dundes. 1992. "Sex Selection and Reproductive Freedom." *Women's Studies International Forum* 15:405-26.

Restivo, Sal. 1988. "Modern Science as a Social Problem." *Social Problems* 35:206-29.

Reunanen, Antti. 1993. "Juhlan Aika Ja Tuonen Hetki" ("The Time of Celebration and the Time of Death"). *Duodecim* 109:2098-103.

Reverby, Susan M. 1987. *Ordered to Care: The Dilemma of American Nursing, 1850-1945.* Cambridge, UK: Cambridge University Press.

Richie, Beth E. 1996. *Compelled to Crime: The Gender Entrapment of Battered Black Women.* New York: Routledge.

Riessman, Catherine Kohler. 1983. "Women and Medicalization: A New Perspective." *Social Policy,* Summer, pp. 3-18.

Riska, Elianne. 1993. "Introduction." Pp. 1-12 in Riska and Wegar.

Riska, Elianne and Katarina Wegar. 1993a. "Women Physicians: A New Force in Medicine?" Pp. 76-93 in Riska and Wegar.

———, eds. 1993b. *Gender, Work and Medicine: Women and the Medical Division of Labor.* Newbury Park, CA: Sage.

Rittenhouse, C. Amanda. 1991. "The Emergence of Premenstrual Syndrome as a Social Problem." *Social Problems* 38:412-25.

Robbins, Cynthia A. and Steven S. Martin. 1993. "Gender, Styles of Deviance, and Drinking Problems." *Journal of Health and Social Behavior* 34:302-21.

Rodriguez-Trias, Helen and Carola Marte. 1995. "Challenges and Possibilities: Women, HIV, and the Health Care System in the 1990s." Pp. 301-21 in Schneider and Stoller.

Rogers, Martha F., Lynne M. Mofenson, and Rovin R. Moseley. 1995. "Reducing the Risk of Perinatal HIV Transmission Through Zidovudine Therapy: Treatment Recommendations and Implications for Perinatal HIV Counseling and Testing." *Journal of the American Medical Women's Association* 50:78-82, 93.

Rogers, Richard G. and Eve Powell-Griner. 1991. "Life Expectancies of Cigarette Smokers and Nonsmokers in the United States." *Social Science and Medicine* 32:1151-59.

Romito, Patrizia and Françoise Hovelaque. 1987. "Changing Approaches in Women's Health: New Insights and New Pitfalls in Prenatal Preventive Care." *International Journal of Health Services* 17:241-58.

Rosenberg, Harriet G. 1984. "The Home Is the Workplace: Hazards, Stress, and Pollutants in the Household." Pp. 219-45 in Chavkin.

Rosenberg, Lynn, Lucile Adams-Campbell, and Julie R. Palmer. 1995. "The Black Women's Health Study: A Follow-Up Study for Causes and Preventions of Illness." *Journal of the American Medical Women's Association* 50:56-63.

Rosenblum, Lisa S., James W. Buehler, Meade W. Morgan, et al. 1993. "Drug Dependence: A Leading Diagnosis in HIV-Infected Women." *Journal of Women's Health* 2:35-40.

Rosenthal, A. M. 1996. "Fighting Female Mutilation." *The New York Times,* April 12, p. A31.

Ross, Catherine E. and Chloe E. Bird. 1994. "Sex Stratification and Health Lifestyle: Consequences for Men's and Women's Perceived Health." *Journal of Health and Social Behavior* 35:161-78.

Rosser, Sue V. 1994. *Women's Health—Missing from U.S. Medicine.* Bloomington: Indiana University Press.

Rossi, Alice S. and Peter Eric Rossi. 1977. "Body Time and Social Time: Mood Patterns by Menstrual Cycle Phase and Day of the Week." *Social Science Research* 6:273-308.

Rotello, Gabriel. 1996. "The Risk in a 'Cure' for AIDS." *The New York Times,* July 14, News of the Week, p. 17.

Roter, Debra, Mack Lipkin, and Audrey Korsgaard. 1991. "Sex Differences in Patients' and Physicians' Communication During Primary Care Medical Visits." *Medical Care* 29:1083-93.

Rothman, Barbara Katz. 1982. *In Labor: Women and Power in the Birthplace.* New York: Norton.

———. 1986. *The Tentative Pregnancy.* New York: Viking.

———. 1989. *Recreating Motherhood: Ideology and Technology in a Patriarchal Society.* New York: Norton.

Roundtable Discussion. 1996. "Health Issures in the Peri- and Postmenopausal Woman: A Multinational Perspective of Women and Their Doctors." *Journal of Women's Health* 5:373-82.

Roxburgh, Susan. 1996. "Gender Differences in Work and Well-Being: Effects of Exposure and Vulnerability." *Journal of Health and Social Behavior* 37:265-77.

Rushing, Beth, Christian Ritter, and Russell P. D. Burton. 1992. "Race Differences in the Effects of Multiple Roles on Health: Longitudinal Evidence from a National Sample of Older Men." *Journal of Health and Social Behavior* 33:126-39.

Ruzek, Sheryl Burt. 1978. *The Women's Health Movement: Feminist Alternatives to Medical Control.* New York: Praeger.

Sabo, Don and David Frederick Gordon, eds. 1995a. *Men's Health and Illness: Gender, Power and the Body.* Thousand Oaks, CA: Sage.

———. 1995b. "Rethinking Men's Health and Illness: The Relevance of Gender Studies." Pp. 1-21 in Sabo and Gordon.

Samson, Michel, Frédérick Libert, Benjamin J. Doranz, et al. 1996. "Resistance to HIV-1 Infection in Caucasian Individuals Bearing Mutant Alleles of the CCR-5 Chemokine Receptor Gene." *Nature* 382(August 22):722-25.

Sandelowski, Margarete. 1993. *With Child in Mind: Studies of the Personal Encounter with Infertility.* Philadelphia: University of Pennsylvania Press.

Santow, Gigi. 1995. "Social Roles and Physical Health: The Case of Female Disadvantage in Poor Countries." *Social Science and Medicine* 40:147-61.

Scambler, Annette and Graham Scambler. 1993. *Menstrual Disorders.* New York: Routledge.

Scheper-Hughes, Nancy. 1992. *Death without Weeping: The Violence of Everyday Life in Brazil.* Berkeley: University of California Press.

———. 1994. "An Essay: 'AIDS and the Social Body.' " *Social Science and Medicine* 39:991-1003.

Scheper-Hughes, Nancy and Margaret M. Lock. 1987. "The Mindful Body: A Prolegomenon to Future Work in Medical Anthropology." *Medical Anthropology Quarterly* n.s. 1:6-41.

Schiebinger, Londa. 1989. *The Mind Has No Sex? Women in the Origins of Modern Science.* Cambridge, MA: Harvard University Press.

Schneider, Beth E. 1992. "AIDS and Class, Gender, and Race Relations." Pp. 19-43 in Huber and Schneider.

Schneider, Beth E. and Nancy E. Stoller, eds. 1995. *Women Resisting AIDS: Feminist Strategies of Empowerment.* Philadelphia: Temple University Press.

Scully, Diana. [1980] 1994. *Men Who Control Women's Health: The Miseducation of Obstetrics and Gynecologists.* New York: Teachers College Press.

Scully, Diana and Pauline Bart. 1973. "A Funny Thing Happened on the Way to the Orifice: Women in Gynecology Textbooks." *American Journal of Sociology* 78:1045-50.

Seals, Brenda F., Michael Hennessy, and Richard L. Sowell. 1996. "Factors Influencing Acceptance and Adherence to Zidovudine Treatment to Prevent Vertical Transmission of HIV." Poster at 11th International Conference on AIDS, Vancouver, Canada.

Seals, Brenda F., Richard L. Sowell, Alice S. Demi, et al. 1995. "Falling through the Cracks: Social Service Concerns of Women Infected with HIV." *Qualitative Health Research* 5:496-515.

Seghal, A., S. Sardena, A. Kumar, et al. 1993. "Role of Male Behavior in Cervical Carcinogenesis among Women with One Lifetime Sexual Partner." *Cancer* 72:1666-69.

Selwyn, Peter A., Patrick G. O'Connor, and Richard S. Schottenfeld. 1995. "Female Drug Users with HIV Infection: Issues for Medical Care and Substance Abuse Treatment." Pp. 241-62 in Minkoff, DeHovitz, and Duerr.

Sen, Amartya K. 1990. "Gender and Cooperative Conflicts." Pp. 123-149 in *Persistent Inequalities: Women and World Development,* edited by Irene Tinker. New York: Oxford University Press.

Shenon, Philip. 1996. "AIDS Epidemic, Late to Arrive, Now Explodes in Populous Asia." *The New York Times,* January 21, Sunday News Section, pp. 1, 8.

Sheon, Amy R., Harold E. Fox, Kenneth C. Rich, et al. 1996. "The Women and Infants Transmission Study (WITS) of Maternal-Infant HIV Transmission: Study Design, Methods, and Baseline Data." *Journal of Women's Health* 5:69-78.

Sherr, Lorraine. 1995. "Psychosocial Aspects of Providing Care for Women with HIV Infection. Pp. 107-23 in Minkoff, DeHovitz, and Duerr.

Sherwin, Susan. 1992. *No Longer Patient: Feminist Ethics and Health Care.* Philadelphia: Temple University Press.

Shilling, Chris. 1993. *The Body and Social Theory.* London: Sage.

Shilts, Randy. 1987. *And the Band Played On: People, Politics and the AIDS Crisis.* Baltimore, MD: Penguin.

Siegel, Karolynn, Martin P. Levine, Charles Brooks, and Rochelle Kern. 1989. "The Motives of Gay Men for Taking or Not Taking the HIV Antibody Test." *Social Problems* 36:368-83.

Simpson, B. Joyce and Ann Williams. 1993. "Caregiving: A Matriarchal Tradition Continues." Pp. 200-11 in Kurth.

Siraisi, Nancy. 1990. *Medieval and Early Renaissance Medicine.* Chicago: University of Chicago Press.

Solomon, D. N. 1961. "Ethnic and Class Differences among Hospitals as Contingencies in Medical Careers." *American Journal of Sociology* 61:463-71.

Sontag, Deborah. 1997. "H.I.V. Testing for Newborns Debated Anew." *The New York Times,* February 10, pp. A1, B6.

Sontag, Susan. 1989. *Illness as Metaphor and AIDS and Its Metaphors.* New York: Doubleday.

Sorensen, Gloria and Lois M. Verbrugge. 1987. "Women, Work, and Health." *American Review of Public Health* 8:235-51.

Sosnowitz, Barbara G. 1995. "AIDS Prevention, Minority Women, and Gender Assertiveness." Pp. 139-61 in Schneider and Stoller.

Sosnowitz, Barbara G. and David R. Kovacs. 1992. "From Burying to Caring: Family AIDS Support Groups." Pp. 131-44 in Huber and Schneider.

Sowell, Richard L., Linda Moneyham, Joyce Guillory, et al. 1997. "Self-Care Activities of Women Infected with Human Immunodeficiency Virus." *Journal of Holistic Nursing Practice* 1:18-26.

Spark, Richard F. 1988. *The Infertile Male: The Clinician's Guide to Diagnosis and Treatment.* New York: Plenum.

Specter, Michael. 1995. "Plunging Life Expectancy Puzzles Russians." *The New York Times,* August 2, p. A1.

Stage, Sarah. 1979. *Female Complaints: Lydia Pinkham and the Business of Women's Medicine.* New York: Norton.

Staples, Robert. 1995. "Health among Afro-American Males." Pp. 121-38 in Sabo and Gordon.

Starr, Paul. 1982. *The Social Transformation of American Medicine.* New York: Basic Books.

Steinem, Gloria. 1978. "If Men Could Menstruate." *MS. Magazine,* October, p. 110.

Steingart, R. M., M. Packer, P. Hamm, et al. 1991. "Sex Differences in the Management of Coronary Artery Disease." *New England Journal of Medicine* 325:226-30.

Steketee, Richard W., R. J. Simonds, E. Abrams, et al. 1996. "Perinatal HIV Transmission Risk and the Effect of Pregnancy or Infant Zidovudine Use in a Multicenter Study, 1994-1995." Abstract, 11th International Conference on AIDS, Vancouver.

Stevens, Patricia E. 1996. "Lesbians and Doctors: Experiences of Solidarity and Domination in Health Care Settings." *Gender & Society* 10:24-41.

Stillion, Judith. 1995. "Premature Death among Males: Extending the Bottom Line of Men's Health." Pp. 46-67 in Sabo and Gordon.

Stokes, J. P., D. J. McKirnan, L. Doll, and R. G. Burzette. 1996. "Female Partners of Bisexual Men: What They Don't Know Might Hurt Them." *Psychology of Women Quarterly* 20:267-84.

Strauss, Anselm, Shizuko Fagerhaugh, Barbara Suczek, and Carolyn Wiener. 1985. *The Social Organization of Medical Work.* Chicago: University of Chicago Press.

Sullivan, Andrew. 1996. "When Plagues End: Notes on the Twilight of an Epidemic." *The New York Times Magazine,* November 10, pp. 52-62, 76-77, 84.

Sundari, T. K. 1994. "The Untold Story: How the Health Care Systems in Developing Countries Contribute to Maternal Mortality." Pp. 173-90 in Fee and Krieger.

Taggart, Lee Ann, Susan L. McCammon, Linda J. Allred, et al. 1993. "Effect of Patient and Physician Gender on Prescriptions for Psychotropic Drugs." *Journal of Women's Health* 2:353-57.

Taylor, Verta. 1995. "Self-Labeling and Women's Mental Health: Postpartum Illness and the Reconstruction of Motherhood." *Sociological Focus* 28:23-47.

Teresi, Dick. 1994. "How to Get a Man Pregnant: My (True) Adventures on the Frontiers of Science." *New York Times Magazine,* November 27, pp. 6, 54.

Tesch, Bonnie J., Helen M. Wood, Amy L. Helwig, and Ann Butler Nattinger. 1995. "Promotion of Women Physicians in Academic Medicine: Glass Ceiling or Sticky Floor?" *Journal of the American Medical Association* 273:1022-25.

Tewksbury, Richard. 1995. "Sexual Adaptations Among Gay Men with HIV." Pp. 222-45 in Sabo and Gordon.

Thoits, Peggy. 1995. "Stress, Coping, and Social Support Processes: Where Are We? What Next?" *Journal of Health and Social Behavior* (Extra issue): 53-79.

Thomas, William I. and Dorothy S. Thomas. 1927. *The Child in America.* New York: Knopf.

Thompson, Becky Wansgaard. 1992. " 'A Way Outa No Way': Eating Problems among African-American, Latina, and White Women." *Gender & Society* 6:546-61.

Todd, Alexandra Dundas. 1989. *Intimate Adversaries: Cultural Conflict Between Doctors and Women Patients.* Philadelphia: University of Pennsylvania Press.

Treichler, Paula A. 1988. "AIDS, Homophobia, and Biomedical Discourse: An Epidemic of Signification." Pp. 31-70 in *AIDS: Cultural Analysis, Cultural Activism,* edited by Douglas Crimp. Cambridge, MA: MIT Press.

———. 1992. "AIDS, HIV, and the Cultural Construction of Reality." Pp. 65-98 in Herdt and Lindenbaum.

Trotter, R. T., A. M. Bowen, J. A. Baldwin, and L. J. Price. 1996. "The Efficacy of Network-Based HIV/AIDS Risk Reduction in Midsize Towns in the United States." *Journal of Drug Issues* 26:591-605.

Turner, Bryan S. 1984. *The Body and Society: Explorations in Social Theory.* London: Basil Blackwell.

———. 1992. *Regulating Bodies: Essays in Medical Sociology.* New York and London: Routledge.

Turner, Heather A., Robert B. Hays and Thomas J. Coates. 1993. "Determinants of Social Support Among Gay Men: The Context of AIDS." *Journal of Health and Social Behavior* 34:37-53.

Turner, R. Jay, Carl F. Grindstaff, and Norma Phillips. 1990. "Social Support and Outcome in Teenage Pregnancy." *Journal of Health and Social Behavior* 31:43-57.

Van Hall, E. V., M. Verdel, and J. Van Der Velden. 1994. " 'Perimenopausal' Complaints in Women and Men: A Comparative Study. *Journal of Women's Health* 3:45-49.

Van Roosmalen, Erica H. and Susan A. McDaniel. 1992. "Adolescent Smoking Intentions: Gender Differences in Peer Context." *Adolescence* 27:87-105.

Veevers, Jean E. and Ellen M. Gee. 1986. "Playing It Safe: Accident Mortality and Gender Roles." *Sociological Focus* 19:349-60.

Verbrugge, Lois M. 1985. "Gender and Health: An Update on Hypotheses and Evidence." *Journal of Health and Social Behavior* 26:156-82.

———. 1986. "Role Burdens and Physical Health of Women and Men." *Women & Health* 11:47-77.

———. 1989a. "The Twain Meet: Empirical Explanations of Sex Differences in Health and Mortality." *Journal of Health and Social Behavior* 30:282-304.

———. 1989b. "Gender, Aging, and Health." Pp. 23-78 in *Aging and Health: Perspectives on Gender, Race, Ethnicity, and Class,* edited by Kyriakos S. Markides. Newbury Park, CA: Sage.

———. 1990. "Pathways of Health and Death." Pp. 41-49 in *Women, Health and Medicine in America,* edited by Rima D. Apple. New York: Garland.

Vertinsky, Patricia. 1990. *The Eternally Wounded Woman: Woman, Doctors and Exercise in the Late Nineteenth Century.* Manchester, UK: Manchester University Press.

Voda, Anne M., Myra Dinnerstein, and Sheryl R. O'Donnell, eds. 1982. *Changing Perspectives on Menopause.* Austin: University of Texas Press.

Vogel, Lise. 1990. "Debating Difference: Feminism, Pregnancy, and the Workplace." *Feminist Studies* 16:9-32.

Waitzkin, Howard. 1983. *The Second Sickness: Contradictions of Capitalist Health Care.* New York: Free Press.

———. 1991. *The Politics of Medical Encounters: How Patients and Doctors Deal with Social Problems.* New Haven, CT: Yale University Press.

Waldron, Ingrid. 1995. "Contributions of Changing Gender Differences in Behavior and Social Roles to Changing Gender Differences in Mortality." Pp. 22-45 in Sabo and Gordon.

Walker, Alice. 1992. *Possessing the Secret of Joy.* New York: Harcourt, Brace, Jovanovich.

Walker, Lenore E. 1984. *The Battered Woman Syndrome.* New York: Springer.

———. 1989. *Terrifying Love: Why Battered Women Kill and How Society Responds.* San Francisco: Harper & Row.

Wallace, Joyce I., Dov Bloch, Robert Whitmore, and Matthew Cushing. 1992. "Fellatio Is a Significant Risk Activity for Acquiring AIDS in New York City

Streetwalking Sex Workers." Poster at 8th International Conference on AIDS, Amsterdam.

Wallace, Joyce I., Felice S. Coral, Ilonna J. Rimm, et al. 1982. "T-Cell Ratios in Homosexuals." Letter. *Lancet*, April 17, p. 908.

Wallace, Joyce I., Joanne Downs, Albert Ott, et al. 1983. "T-Cell Ratios in New York City Prostitutes." Letter. *Lancet*, January 1/8:58-59.

Wallis, Lila. 1994. "Why a Curriculum on Women's Health?" Pp. 13-26 in Dan.

Walsh, Mary Roth. 1977. *"Doctors Wanted: No Women Need Apply": Sexual Barriers in the Medical Profession, 1835-1975*. New Haven, CT: Yale University Press.

———. 1990. "Women in Medicine Since Flexner." *New York State Journal of Medicine* 90:302-08.

Warshaw, Carole. 1989. "Limitations of the Medical Model in the Case of Battered Women." *Gender & Society* 3:506-17.

———. 1996. "Domestic Violence: Changing Theory, Changing Practice." *Journal of the American Medical Women's Association* 51:87-91.

Wawer, M. J., C. Podhisita, U. Kanungsukkasem, et al. 1996. "Origins and Working Conditions of Female Sex Workers in Thailand: Consequences of Social Context for HIV Transmission." *Social Science and Medicine* 42:453-62.

Weisman, Carol S. and Martha Ann Teitelbaum. 1985. "Physician Gender and the Physician-Patient Relationship: Recent Evidence and Relevant Questions." *Social Science and Medicine* 20:1119-27.

Weitz, Rose. 1992. *Life with AIDS*. New Brunswick, NJ: Rutgers University Press.

———. 1996. *The Sociology of Health, Illness, and Health Care: A Critical Approach*. Belmont, CA: Wadsworth.

Wenger, Nanette K. 1994. "Coronary Heart Disease in Women: Gender Differences in Diagnostic Evaluation." *Journal of the American Medical Women's Association* 49:181-85.

Wermuth, Laurie, Jennifer Ham, and Rebecca L. Robbins. 1992. "Women Don't Wear Condoms: AIDS Risk Among Sexual Partners of IV Drug Users." Pp. 72-94 in Huber and Schneider.

West, Candace. 1984. *Routine Complications: Troubles with Talk between Doctors and Patients*. Bloomington: Indiana University Press.

White, Evelyn C., ed. 1990. *The Black Women's Health Book: Speaking for Ourselves*. Seattle, WA: Seal Press.

Whitmore, Robert, Joyce I. Wallace, Dov Bloch, and Priscilla Alexander. 1996. "HIV Testing Rates in New York City Streetwalkers Have Declined." Poster at 11th International Conference on AIDS, Vancouver.

Wilcox, Allen, Rolv Skjaerven, and Pierre Buekens. 1995. "Birth Weight and Perinatal Mortality: A Comparison of the United States and Norway." *Journal of the American Medical Association* 273:709-11.

Wilkinson, Doris Y. and Marvin B. Sussman. 1987. *Alternative Health Maintenance and Healing Systems for Families*. New York: Haworth.

Williams, Christine L. 1989. *Gender Differences at Work: Women and Men in Nontraditional Occupations*. Berkeley: University of California Press.

———. 1992. "The Glass Escalator: Hidden Advantages for Men in the 'Female' Professions." *Social Problems* 39:253-67.

———. 1995. *Still a Man's World: Men Who Do "Women's Work."* Berkeley: University of California Press.

Williams, Linda S. 1988. " 'It's Going to Work for Me.' Responses to Failures of IVF." *Birth* 15:153-56.

Wilson, Margo and Martin Daly. 1985. "Competitiveness, Risk Taking, and Violence: The Young Male Syndrome." *Ethology and Sociobiology* 6:59-73.

Wilson, Robert. 1966. *Feminine Forever.* New York: M. Evans.

Wingard, Deborah L., Barbara A. Cohn, Piera M. Cirillo, et al. 1992. "Gender Differences in Self-Reported Heart Disease Morbidity: Are Intervention Opportunities Missed for Women?" *Journal of Women's Health* 1:201-8.

Wood, Connie Shear. 1979. *Human Sickness and Health: A Biocultural View.* Palo Alto, CA: Mayfield.

World Health Organization. 1995. *Women's Health: Improve our Health, Improve the World.* Position paper, Fourth World Conference on Women, Beijing, China.

Wright, D. C., R. R. Redfield, D. S. Burke, and J. L. Rhoads. 1987. "Chronic Vaginal Candidiasis in Women with Human Immunodeficiency Virus Infection." *Journal of the American Medical Association* 257:3105-7.

Wright, Lawrence. 1996. "Silent Sperm." *The New Yorker,* January 15, pp. 42-55.

Wright, Peter and Andrew Treacher. 1982. *The Problem of Medical Knowledge: Examining the Social Construction of Medicine.* Edinburgh, UK: Edinburgh University Press.

Yankauskas, Ellen. 1990. "Primary Female Syndromes: An Update." *New York State Journal of Medicine* 90:295-302.

Yedidia, Michael J., Carolyn A. Berry, and Judith K. Barr. 1996. "Changes in Physicians' Attitudes Towards AIDS During Residency Training: A Longitudinal Study of Medical School Graduates." *Journal of Health and Social Behavior* 37:179-91.

Yllö, Kersti. 1984. "The Status of Women, Marital Equality, and Violence Against Wives. *Journal of Family Issues* 5:307-20.

Ziegler, R. G. 1993. "Migration Patterns and Breast Cancer Risk in Asian-American Women." *Journal of the National Cancer Institute* 85:1819-27.

Zimmerman, Mary K. 1987. "The Women's Health Movement: A Critique of Medical Enterprise and the Position of Women." Pp. 442-72 in *Analyzing Gender,* edited by Beth B. Hess and Myra Marx Ferree. Newbury Park, CA: Sage.

Zita, Jacquelyn. 1988. "The Premenstrual Syndrome: "Dis-easing" the Female Cycle." *Hypatia* 3:77-99.

———. 1993. "Heresy in the Female Body: The Rhetorics of Menopause." Pp. 59-78 in Callahan.

Cushing, M., 91

Dahl, C., 53
Daly, M., 23
Dan, A. J., 12, 54, 98
Danner, S. W., 83
Darrow, S. L., 26
Daum, M., 74
Davis, K., 4, 41, 51, 66
Davis, M. D., 76, 82
Dean, M., 73
Death:
    immediate cause of, 17
    proximate cause of, 17
Death dips, 30-32, 33
    Chinese astrology and, 31-32
    Christmas, 31
    definition of, 30
    Easter, 31
    Harvest Moon Festival, 31
    Passover, 31
    post-birthday, 31
    Yom Kippur, 31
DeCherney, A. H., 21
DeCiantis, M. L., 47
Deeb, L. C., 15
Delaney, J., 57
Delany, S. R., 87
Demi, A. S., 83, 84, 92
de Villiers, E. M., 53
Diagnosis, politics of, 8
Diamond, T., 39
Diaz, Y. E., 77
Dickinson, C., 28
Dickson, G. L., 64
DiClemente, R. J., 71, 75
Dinnerstein, M., 13, 69
Dixon-Mueller, R., 18
Doctor-nurse-patient relationship, 8, 100
    power differences in, 9, 40-41
    See also Feminist health care; Physicians;
        Nurses; Patients
Doll, L. S., 71, 73
Domestic violence. *See* Battering
Donovan, J. E., 24
Doranz, B. J., 73
Douglas, M., 58
Downs, J., 70
Dowsett, G. W., 76
Doyal, L., 12
Drachman, V., 38, 53
Draper, E., 20
Dual-career marriages, double-shift for women
    in, 28, 33

Dubler, N. N., 81, 92
Duerr, A. C., 77, 81
Dugger, C. W., 25, 34
Dunlap, D. W., 78, 86, 92, 93, 96
Dying, gendered patterns of, 30-32, 33

Eberstein, I. W., 15
Eckenrode, J., 28
Ecosocial theory, 16
Egan, A., 13, 55, 59, 67, 69
Egan, T., 36
Ehrenreich, B., 12, 54, 65
Eiston, M. A., 53
Ekstrom, B., 64
El Dareer, A., 26
Eli Lilly and Company, 97
Engholm, G., 53
English, D., 12, 54, 65
Epstein, A. M., 47
Erni, J. N., 83, 84
Estrogen replacement therapy, 62, 68
    as routine, 97
    breast cancer risk from, 30, 63, 97
    dangers of, 63
    endometrial cancer risk from, 63
    heart disease prevention from, 63, 68
    osteoporosis prevention from, 63, 68
Ettorre, E., 9, 27
Etzel, S. I., 51
European Collaborative Study, 80
Evatt, B. L., 82

Faden, R. R., 54, 81
Fagerhaugh, S., 39
Farberow, N. L., 18
Farhi, M. S., 92
Farnsworth, P., 92
Farrell, J., 34
Farrell, M. P., 26
Fausto-Sterling, A., 12, 60, 69
Featherstone, M., 12
Federman, D., 54
Fee, E., 6, 8, 12
Feldman, K. A., 31
Female physiology:
    as pathology, 51
Feminist health care, 11, 98-102
    and creating expert knowledge on women's
        health, 101
    and creating interdisciplinary women's
        health specialty, 101
    as context-based, 99
    focus of, 98

Kanungsukkasem, U., 72
Kashima, Y., 34
Kasl, S. V., 31
Kassler, W. J., 84
Kauppinen-Toropainen, K., 53
Kay, B. J., 39
Kearney-Cooke, A., 24
Keller, E. F., 12, 53, 98
Kelly, J. A., 74, 77, 78
Kelly, P. J., 83, 84, 92
Kemp, A. A., 28
Kemper, T. D., 60
Kennedy, M. B., 77
Kern, R., 79
Kessler, R. C., 36, 52
Kimmel, M., 76
King, D., 74
King, E. W., 31
Kippax, S., 76
Kitagawa, E. M., 23
Klaukka, T., 9, 27
Kliewer, E. V., 15, 53
Klinge, I., 63
Kloske, B., 34
Knight, C., 55, 56
Kobasa, S. C., 28
Koch, L., 22, 34
Koeske, R. D., 57, 60, 69
Kolata, G., 36, 72
Koos, E. L., 1
Kopriva, P., 51
Koreck, M. T., 74
Korsgaard, A., 46
Korvick, J. A., 82
Kovacs, D. R., 84
Kramer, L., 83
Kranczer, S., 14, 15, 23
Kreuter, M. W., 9, 45
Krieger, N., 6, 8, 12, 16
Kristiansen, C. M., 12
Kumar, A., 53
Kurz, D., 29, 43

Lachenbruch, P. A., 3
Lai, G., 28
Lammi, J., 53
Landesman, S., 92
Laqueur, T., 12
Larson, M. S., 53
Lasker, J. N., 34
Late Luteal Phase Dysphoric Disorder, 59
Latour, B., 53
Laumann, E. O., 91
Lavin, B., 50

Laws, S., 13, 55, 58, 59, 60, 67, 69
Lay healers, 36
Lazarus, E., 34, 41
Lear, D., 92
Leite, M., 74
Lennane, K. J., 69
Lennane, R. J., 69
Lennon, M. C., 28, 34
Leonard, J. M., 83
Lesbian AIDS Project, 77
Leslie, C., 36
Levenson, A., 29
Levesque-Lopman, L., 62
Levine, C., 79, 80, 81, 82
Levine, M. P., 76, 77, 79, 91
Levy, K. B., 58
Lewin, E., 12
Lewis, D. K., 73, 74
Lewis, J., 63
Li, J., 19
Libert, F., 73
Lieberman, E., 23, 34
Life expectancy rates, 15, 16
 African American, 14
 low social status and, 14-15
 See also Life expectancy rates (female); Life expectancy rates (male)
Life expectancy rates (female):
 access to childbirth medical care and, 32
 access to prenatal medical care and, 32
 Africans, 16
 Asians, 16
 Europeans, 16
 for U.S. white, 14
 in developed countries, 16
 in developing countries, 16
 Latin American, 16
 North American, 16
 of former USSR, 16
 of Oceania, 16
Life expectancy rates (male):
 Africans, 16
 Asians, 16
 Europeans, 16
 for U.S. African American, 14, 23
 for U.S. white, 14
 in developed countries, 16
 in developing countries, 16
 Latin Americans, 16
 North American, 16
 of former USSR, 16
 of Oceania, 16
Lightfoot-Klein, H., 25, 26
Lillard, L. A., 28
Lindenbaum, S., 40

Menstrual cycle:
  and subordination of women, 57, 67
  exercise and, 57
  medicalizing, 58-59
  non-Western cultural model of, 55-56
  Profet's theory on function of, 57
  scientific view of, 56
  seen as illness, 55, 67
  social construction of, 57-58
Menstrual taboos, women's oppression and, 56
Merrick, J. C., 34
Mertz, D., 91
Messner, M., 4, 24, 27
Meyer, D. L., 46
Miall, C. E., 34
Michaels, S., 91
Michelis, M. A., 70
Midwives, 38
  resurgence of, 49
  supplemental care by, 41
  versus obstetricians, 49
  See also Nurse midwives
Minichiello, V., 92
Minkoff, H., 82
Mishler, E. G., 2, 9, 12, 40
Mitchell, E. O., 101
Mofenson, L. M., 92
Moldow, G., 7, 37, 48, 53
Moneyham, L., 84, 92
Monson, R. R., 23, 34
Morantz, R. M., 53
Morantz-Sanchez, R. M., 38, 53
Morbidity rates, 15
  adolescence/young adulthood and
    gendered patterns of, 22-26
  adulthood and gendered patterns of, 26-27
  assessing, 17
  childbirth/infancy and gendered patterns
    of, 18-19
  cultural factors and, 18
  dying and gendered patterns of, 30-32
  government financial support for
    research/treatment and, 18
  health care institutions'/agencies' policies
    and, 18
  health care providers' behavior and, 18
  infertility and gendered patterns of, 19-22
  old age and gendered patterns of, 30
  social factors and, 18
  work and family and gendered patterns of,
    27-30
Morgan, J. H., 36
Morgan, M. W., 73
Mortality rates, 15
  cultural factors and, 18

government financial support for
  research/treatment and, 18
health care institutions'/agencies' policies
  and, 18
health care providers' behavior and, 18
social factors and, 18
Moseley, R. R., 92
Muller, C., 12, 17, 34
Muncy, R., 48
Musico, M., 74

Nachtigall, L. B., 30, 63
Nachtigall, L. E., 30, 63
Nachtigall, R. D., 21
Nam, C. B., 15
National Coalition for Women's Mental Health,
  61
National Institutes of Health, 50, 75
  Office of Alternative Medicine, 36
  Office of Women's Health Research, 50
Native American healers:
  medical community's view of, 7
Native medicine, 36
  in China, 36
  in India, 36
Nattinger, A. B., 53
Navarro, M., 71, 85
Nechas, E., 70, 91
Neigus, A., 72, 78
Newman, K. L., 24
Nicolosi, A., 74
Nightingale, Florence, 38
Norlock, F. E., 36, 52
Norman, D. K., 24
Nosek, M. A., 50, 100
Notzer, N., 53
Novello, A. C., 83
Nsiah-Jefferson, L., 20
Nurse midwives, 7, 39
Nurse practitioners, 7, 9, 38, 39, 66-67, 100
Nurses, 52
  African American, 39
  defining role of, 38-40
  Hispanic, 39
  licensed practical, 39
  male, 39
  registered, 39
  supplemental care by, 41, 98
  See also Nurse midwives; Nurse
    practitioners; Nursing profession
Nursing profession:
  racially stratified hierarchy within, 39
  stratification by education/degree, 39
  versus medical profession, 35

Judith Lorber is Professor Emerita of Sociology at Brooklyn College and the Graduate School, City University of New York, where she was first Coordinator of the Women's Studies Certificate Program. She has published numerous articles on women as health care workers and patients and on sociological aspects of the new procreative technologies. She is author of *Paradoxes of Gender* (1994) and of *Women Physicians: Careers, Status and Power* (1984). She was founding editor of *Gender & Society*, official publication of Sociologists for Women in Society, and, with Susan A. Farrell, coedited a collection of papers from that journal, *The Social Construction of Gender* (Sage, 1991). She was Chair of the Sex and Gender Section of the American Sociological Association in 1993 and received the 1996 ASA Jessie Bernard Career Award.